W9-BDZ-266

GOVERNORS STATE UNIVERSITY LIBRARY

3 1611 00095 8428

DATE DUE

10/06/05	IL: 11365878	
05/17/06	IL: 17979 888	
3-2-07	IL: 26375154	
6/1/07	ILLINET	
7-29-08	IL: 43247502	
10-4-8	IL: 45081081	
11/19/08	ILLINET	
10-26-9	IL: 56860721	
5-25-10	IL: 6405706	
8/6/11	IL: 82699517	
5-9-13	IL: 101767561	
7/3/13	IL: 104145064	
9/24/15	ILIS 1647239	
APR 05 2024		223084769

Demco, Inc. 38-293

Three Weeks in Spring

GOVERNORS STATE UNIVERSITY
UNIVERSITY PARK
IL 60466

Also by Robert B. Parker

Three Weeks in Spring ⌒

by Joan H. Parker
& Robert B. Parker

Houghton Mifflin Company Boston 1978

UNIVERSITY LIBRARY
GOVERNORS STATE UNIVERSITY
PARK FOREST SOUTH, ILL.

For Jude. She made it better.

Copyright © 1978 by Joan H. and Robert B. Parker

*All rights reserved. No part of this work may be reproduced
or transmitted in any form by any means, electronic or
mechanical, including photocopying and recording, or by
any information storage or retrieval system, without
permission in writing from the publisher.*

Library of Congress Cataloging in Publication Data

Parker, Joan H
   Three weeks in spring.

    1. Breast — Cancer — Biography. 2. Parker,
Joan H.   I. Parker, Robert B., 1932–   joint
author.   II. Title.
RC280.B8P29   362.1'9'699449   77–12396
ISBN 0–395–26282–8

Printed in the United States of America
P 10 9 8 7 6 5 4 3 2 1

Check Out Receipt

Marion Carnegie Library (MRNP-ZCA
)
618-993-5935
www.marioncarnegielibrary.org/

Friday, January 12, 2024 12:01:08
 PM
10041

Title: Three weeks in spring
Due: 1/26/2024

You just saved $25.00 by using yo
ur library. You have saved $25.00
 this past year and $9,501.51 sin
ce you began using the library!

Check out MCL's Video Game collec
tion on the library's top and bot
tom floors!

280
.B8
P29

Prologue ⌒

He couldn't remember when he hadn't loved her. It was the fundamental condition of his life. It seemed as if he had been born loving her. But, in fact, he hadn't loved her until he was eighteen and they met at college. She was old family, good manners, and what does your father do. He was at some momentary place between poet and thug. They were drawn together and sustained by a shared sense of humor that developed over the years into a complex and delicate instrument of communication, a ritual of relationship, inviolate and enduring.

Twenty-five years after they first met, and eighteen years after they married, her cancerous left breast was removed, and when she came out of the anesthesia and saw him standing at the foot of the bed in the green hospital room neither of them knew if the cancer had spread and she was going to die.

She said, "Easy come, easy go."

He said, "Look at the bright side, you can probably get bras at half price."

She smiled and nodded and closed her eyes and went back to sleep and he stood in the quiet room with the television set making antic motions but no sound and watched her sleep.

Three Weeks in Spring

Chapter 1 ⌒

Friday, April 11

IT BEGAN LATE, Dave and Dan in bed, a steak poised on the grill and half a gallon of Gallo Rhine Garten chilling in the refrigerator; the house they'd built mostly themselves was gleaming and orderly the way she always put it before she went to bed, and she was in the bathtub while he, showered and shaved, strolled about in his blue bathrobe with the sleeves cut off, saying lascivious things to her through the nearly closed door of the bathroom.

She always took a long time in the bath before they made love and he always waited impatiently. She shaved her legs and then lathered and shaved under her arms. As her hands brushed her left breast she felt a lump. She denied it. She stopped. Felt it again. *What the hell is this? It's the weights.* She had been firming the backs of her arms with two small dumbbells that he had bought her at Sears and she thought, *this is new muscle, that's all, I'll have one on the other side.* She felt it again. It was there and it didn't feel like a muscle. It didn't feel like anything she could define. She felt the other side. If *there's a lump on the right breast I'll know it's okay. Please God let there be a lump there too.* There wasn't one there.

She could hear him walking around, putting two wine glasses in the freezer to chill, talking to the dog. She could hear the dog's footsteps. His claws clack-clack on the kitchen floor in a sound so familiar she didn't remember hearing it before. *This is impossible,* she thought, *this cannot be happening to me. I'm sitting up in the tub and I'm feeling my left breast and there's something there and it could be a cancerous tumor, but I'm not doing it right. I'll lie on the floor like you're supposed to and I'll elevate the shoulder blades somewhat and I'll go over the breast with my fingers flat in a circular motion section by section like the face of a clock.* She did this. The lump was there and she felt the sick panic come over her in waves like nausea. She sweated and fought off the panic.

"If you don't get out of there pretty soon I'm going to make a move on the goddamned dog," he said through the door.

"In a minute." The panic was there, heavy on her chest, and she had to have more time to fight it off. *I'm a pessimist,* she said to herself, *I always assume the worst. Eighty-five percent of tumors are nonmalignant. And there's Ace waiting for me and I'll put this aside. I will make love to him and I will put this aside. There are all sorts of cysts and benign tumors and that's probably what I've got.* And she learned the first thing that she was to learn in these three weeks. She learned that she could put aside her panic and deal with the things that were coming along in the order that they needed to be dealt with.

She toweled dry and brushed her teeth and put a touch of perfume at her throat and went in to make love to her husband.

In bed with him, her arms around him, she pressed her open hands against his back. He was a big man who lifted weights and his back was as broad and solid as a steamer trunk. The solidity of his physical presence had always seemed to her the visible embodiment of his commitment and now it made her sad to think how little avail that physical strength was if the lump was bad. *But the commitment,* she thought, *the commitment is there.* *Even if the lump is bad, the commitment is there,* and she pressed her hands as hard as she could against the mass of his back and felt his weight against her and kissed him and thought no more of the tumor for a while.

At two that morning they sat at their kitchen counter and ate steak and drank the chilled white wine, as they had a hundred times before.

"You won't tell about how I drink cold white wine with steak, will you?" he said. "We could never eat at the Ritz again."

"It's not the temperature that will get you in trouble," she said. "It's the quantity." She pretended to scratch under her left arm. The lump was still there. The knowledge of it never left her, but she had put it into a spot in her mind, off the main track, isolated there like a frightful star, bright but remote. *I must be crazy,* she thought. *I can't be sitting here with a lump in my breast. At least he didn't discover it while we were in bed and say, 'What's this lump in your breast?'*

Maybe, she thought, *I should tell him. I could say, 'Hey, you know what? I have this lump in my breast and I'm really afraid I have breast cancer.'* But she couldn't. She couldn't say it out loud. That would make it real. Much realer than it was now. Much scarier. And to see it in his face, reflected back at her. The fear made tangible in his eyes and the set of his mouth. No, it was better to be quiet. Not so much to spare him. To spare her.

He poured the last of the wine and raised his glass to her.

"Here's looking at you, kid," he said in a barely recognizable imitation of Humphrey Bogart.

"That is probably the most terrible Humphrey Bogart imitation I've ever heard," she said.

"That's not what all the co-eds say," he said.

"What do the co-eds say?"

"They say I'm such good tail that it doesn't matter."

"They're wrong," she said.

He laughed out loud. "Let's go to bed," he said.

And they did.

And she slept.

Chapter 2 ~⌒

Saturday, April 12

THE MORNING was bright spring. The lump felt smaller than it had Friday night. Saturday afternoon it felt bigger than it had Saturday morning. She went through the weekend feeling the lump in her breast, touching it, touching it. Talking to herself. *It'll go away. It's the kind that changes like that, it will be gone soon. I take good care of myself.*

She did take good care of herself. She was regular in going to the doctor for Pap smears. She was careful about her eating. She rode her Exercycle three miles a day. She'd given up smoking more than a year ago. She cared about her body and was proud of it. *My mother did not have breast cancer,* she thought. *I am not menopausal. The odds are with me. It is just unlikely that this will be a malignant mass.*

The front yard was mushy. The frost had melted and the last traces of snow were gone, except in the recesses where the trailing roses ran along the low fieldstone fence they had built. The bright April sun shone on the debris of winter: dead grass, MacDonald's wrappers, the sports section of the *Globe,* crumpled and water-stained under the willow tree. There were dog droppings and a dead bird decomposing near the maple tree. The brick walk that they had laid in sand together three summers ago had buckled and needed to be reset here and there.

She said, "Ace, are you going to do the yard today?"

"Maybe, after I read the paper."

"You and your goddamned paper," she said.

"Saturdays," he said, "I like to read the paper and drink my coffee. The yard's not going anywhere."

"It's a goddamned mess," she said.

"Well, go clean it up. You want it cleaned, you do it. When I want it cleaned I'll do it. I don't mind it."

The bastard. That's how he always got her. She was compulsive about the yard and the house and he wasn't. They were too liberated to talk of man's work and woman's work. He cooked. She painted the house. She couldn't say, "But yard work is your job." They were way past that and sometimes she looked back a little wistfully to when they weren't.

"Besides, the yard's too wet for raking. You'll tear up all the grass."

"Shit," she said. She put on his blue warm-up jacket, six sizes too big, that said TENNESSEE TECH STAFF on it, and went out and cleaned up the yard savagely.

Smug bastard. I'm out here raking the yard with maybe goddamned breast cancer and he's in there reading 'Broom Hilda.' But of course he doesn't know. It's not like I've told him. You'd think one of the boys would come out, maybe give me a hand with the yard. They don't care. They'd rather stay in and fight with each other. I'm the only one that cares about this house.

She could feel the tears begin to form.

Not that way, Joan, for God's sake not that way. Don't get into the horror of self-pity. You'll get in too deep, you won't be able to get out. You've got to stay out of that, Joan. But alone, oh God, it's hard alone. But it's harder if they know. I can spare them that until I have to. I can spare me that. Don't lie to yourself, it's me that I'm sparing. I'm not Nancy Noble. I don't want him looking at me thinking of the terror that might be ahead of us. The horror that might be ahead of us.

She went and opened the back door. He wasn't there. She went in. She heard the shower running in the downstairs bath. He was in there, showering, singing "The Impossible Dream" in his harsh New England voice and flatting badly on the high notes.

She stuck her head in the bathroom door. "When you get through with your shower," she said, "could you take a minute and get rid of a dead bird for me, or haven't you finished your paper yet?"

He didn't like having his singing interrupted. "Yeah," he said. "I'll be out in a few minutes."

It was almost twenty minutes before he did come out. The bird was in the way. She wanted to rake where it was but she couldn't stand to pick it up. He came out with his hair still wet and his shirt off in the raw spring air. *He really ought to lose twenty pounds,* she thought. He got a shovel from the garage and scooped the decaying carcass of the bird from the lawn and took it out back and flicked it into the woods. He put the shovel back in the garage and went back in the house without comment.

She put her hand inside the jacket and felt her breast again; the lump was there. As it had been since last night.

It was there all afternoon while he watched the season's first ball game on network television and the boys had a long argument over whether they'd go to the movies or not. She tired of the lawn and went in and lay down in the bedroom and tried to take a nap and tried to keep the thoughts of her breast off in that cold bright spot in the upper corner of her consciousness. If she could keep it there, balanced, and still, it wouldn't sweep down and swamp her. And she managed. She kept it there carefully, the way you would carry a very full glass, not spilling a drop. The knowledge of her lump was like that and she was able to do it, to keep it up there, and still, and even take a nap.

When she woke with a soggy feeling and a sense of unspecified apprehension he was in the kitchen making a venison meat loaf for the boys' supper and drinking Miller Lite from the can. Lying on the bed she could hear the pop top come off the can. He drank too much. What was she apprehensive about. *Oh God, yes. The breast. What if it were bad, would he drink more? Maybe he wouldn't be able to cope and he'd jump into a bottle, as they said on the soap operas. Or a beer can. If he couldn't handle this it would kill him. He had to be able to handle things. He needed that for his sense of himself. What if he couldn't? But he always had — some tough things too. But, Jesus Christ, nothing like this. What if he went under and she died and the boys . . .*

She got up abruptly and went to the kitchen; the TV set on the counter showed the waning innings of the ball game. He was crumbing oatmeal bread in the blender.

"We have to be ready to leave at seven-thirty," she said. Her voice was flat and unloving, grayed by the annoyance of the afternoon. She felt like fighting with him. He nodded without speaking. *What the hell is he annoyed about?* she thought. *He's been in here reading the paper, watching the ball game, drinking his goddamned beer, and I've been out in the yard with goddamned breast cancer maybe, raking my ass off.*

"You hear me?" she said.

"Yup."

"You don't feel like answering me."

"I nodded," he said.

She made a cup of instant coffee without saying anything else.

At seven-thirty she wasn't ready and he waited without comment while she got ready. She was never ready on time. They went with the Marshes to a great large party in a restored colonial house with more than a hundred invited guests. It was more interesting than it might otherwise have been because of several factors. The house was fascinating, perhaps fifteen or twenty rooms, restored and furnished by people who cared about the task and knew about the period. For another thing the Parkers hadn't been invited.

The Marshes had been invited and had convinced them they should come. In a party this size who would care about two more? And they could have fun making a lot of private humor among all those people. It was a different thing to be doing on a Saturday night and Joan was able to think about the party enough so as not to think about her breast.

In all this mob, she thought at one point, *I'm the only one who knows. What if I stopped someone and told them: 'Hello, I have a lump in my breast that might be malignant.' Wouldn't that pick things up.*

She smoked occasionally that night, though she hadn't for a year, bumming three cigarettes during the evening, and she was buoyed, as she always was, by the excitement of the party, the challenge of conversation, the pleasure of making people laugh. She was good at interacting and she knew it. It was one of the things she was proud of. He did not like small talk. She always said his only outstanding social skill was ending a conversation.

"I prefer to think that I do not suffer fools gladly," he said, and patted her covertly on the backside.

"Mr. Warm," she said. "You and John are about as much fun at a party as Charlie Manson."

"Or the Masque of the Red Death."

"The what?"

"It's a story by Poe, you know, there's a party . . ."

She yawned elaborately.

"Screw," he said.

They left the party near midnight and went home, with the Marshes. She was elevated. Elated by the contact and the slightly illegitimate nature of their attendance, by the pleasures of being with the Marshes, friends for ten years with whom they spent three Saturday nights out of five and whom they saw nearly every day.

It's just a simple damned cyst, she said to herself as she lay in bed poking at her breast, feeling the lump in the dark while he snored beside her in the bed. *It's just a cyst.*

Chapter 3 ~

Sunday, April 13

SHE PLANNED. Saturday she had raked the front yard. Sunday she raked the back. And while she raked she planned her approach to the lump in her breast. *Tomorrow is the day I do something,* she thought. *Now what am I going to do? I teach Mondays from nine to one so the doctor appointment has to be in the afternoon.* She got the tines of the rake caught in the branches of a small azalea and yanked at it savagely. From the house she could hear Dan scream at David. *Why in hell doesn't Ace do something about that? Why in hell doesn't he make them stop?* There was a thunderous clattering from the house. *Don't run up and down stairs,* she murmured to herself.

When shall I call Dr. Barry? Who would be around on a Sunday? Just the answering service. They couldn't make an appointment. Just like the kids, she thought, *only get sick on weekends when no one's around. Have to call Dr. Barry from school for an appointment. I'll do that tomorrow.* And, as she raked, she phrased how she'd do it. How casually she would phrase her request for an appointment. *'I'm very sorry to bother you,'* she would say, with a lot of those cultured overtones she'd learned from her early years as a service representative with the telephone company, *'I'm very sorry to bother you, but I believe I've found a lump in my left breast. Probably it isn't anything, but would it be possible for the doctor to see me?'*

In the woods behind the house a cardinal swept down to the ground, picked something up and flew off. *A cardinal. For heaven's sake. I haven't seen a cardinal since about third grade.*

Of course if they gave her a hard time then she would scream at them: *'Jesus Christ,'* she would yell, *'if you don't see me I'm going to put a gun to my head.'* She rehearsed her phone call over and over and over, saying it to herself again and again. *'I'm very sorry to bother you, but I believe I've found a lump in my left breast.'*

The cardinal came back, brilliant and flitting in the new-leafed shadows of the spring woods. She remembered the little girl in the third grade on the nature walk that they had to take every week, and how she'd had to hold hands with Billy Van Bueren as they went two by two and the teacher named birds and plants that they passed. Billy Van Bueren, she remembered, had fallen on hard times. His parents had died and he'd gone to an orphanage or a foster home, or whatever. But that had been later and, that day, looking at the cardinal and holding hands, they hadn't thought of things like that.

Monday, April 14

She called Dr. Barry's office from school and got squeezed in for a Monday night appointment. She told her husband and her sons that it was a routine check on some minor vaginal bleeding that she'd experienced occasionally before. He said something about front end trouble and they both smiled at the joke. Like all of their humor it was a several-layered thing, making fun not only of her, but of him as the kind of person who would say that, and of the clichéd phrase and the kind of people who would use it. And they both knew all of the layers and smiled at them all without a pause to think about it.

"But it will be all right, won't it?" Dan said. He was the youngest of them and had not yet acquired much ability to mask his feelings. David had already learned to internalize. Too much so, she sometimes thought, like his father. She was more like Dan. She felt and she allowed the feelings to show.

"It's nothing," she said. "I've had it before. Most ladies do at one time or another."

When she left at eight-fifteen the boys were doing homework and Ace was cleaning up the kitchen. The appliances were poppy-red, and in the brick wall at the far end Ace had set a stained-glass window that she'd found in an antique shop in New Hampshire. It was a beautiful kitchen, the collaboration of their imagination and their hands.

It was eight-thirty when she got to Barry's office. It was quarter of eleven when she got in to see the doctor. Waiting there was one of the most traumatizing things she did before surgery. No one had ever seen the office so busy; it was unusual on a Monday night. "We're really awfully sorry you ladies have to wait so long." Joan's nervousness expressed itself in diarrhea. *I may die of terminal diarrhea before I get in the office,* she thought. Between sieges she read a magazine article on redecorating the bathroom. *Appropriate,* she thought. *But amazing. I'm sitting here getting ideas for a new bathroom décor while waiting for an examination for breast cancer. There's the little part of my brain that separates out the terror, and the rest responds to whatever the environment dishes up.* She looked at the magazine pictures of a gallery wall treatment in a bathroom, and stored it away. *We'll do that. That's really a neat idea.*

When they ushered her into the examining room it was very

lonely. Barry wasn't there yet. She took off her blouse and bra and folded them neatly on the chair, the blouse modestly covering the bra. She put on the paper johnny that gapped open in the front and seemed to emphasize her nakedness. She wondered as she always did at the doctor's why they bothered. *The only thing it conceals is my back. If someone's a shoulder blade freak I've got him thwarted.* She always hated sitting there alone on the table with the stirrups, waiting to be examined. But this was worse. Much worse. It was a very, very alone feeling.

Barry came in. A nice guy, friendly, quite distinguished-looking, also very tired at nearly eleven at night. "Doctor," Joan said, "I'm very sorry but I've got to know what this thing is."

"I know," he said. He pressed his fingertips gently on the surface of her breasts, kneading and prodding both breasts, touching the lump in the left and then beginning to feel it, and all around it.

"Does this hurt? Does this hurt? Any discomfort there?"

"I don't think any of it hurts," she said. "But I've been thinking about it so much I can't tell anymore. I'm so aware of it, you know?"

"Yes," he said. "Does this hurt?"

She shook her head. He moved his fingertips in a small semicircle around the lump in her left breast. The Muzak played softly above her head. Other than that it was quiet. Dr. Barry was a physically reassuring man. Logical-looking. He finished examining her breasts and said, "Well you're not imagining something. There's a lump in your left breast okay."

Joan said, "Uh-huh. What do you think it might be?" *So calm, so matter of fact. Might it be a malignant tumor? Might you have to cut off my boob?*

Barry said, "I want to try something." The nurse gave him a long hypodermic needle. "This won't hurt," the nurse said. "It looks bad but it isn't." And it wasn't. Barry probed for a long time at the lump in Joan's left breast. *What the hell is he doing, is he trying to move the lump? Is he trying to figure out how big it is?* Dr. Barry was the kind of man who answered such questions, but she didn't ask. She wanted only that he be done and tell her it was nothing. A simple bit of fatty tissue, a small sebaceous cyst that could be excised on an outpatient basis.

He took the needle out and said, "You know, I would really be a lot happier if I could aspirate that."

"What's that mean?" Joan asked.

"If I could have gotten a little fluid out, we'd know a lot better," he said. "Then we could inject a little fluid in and it would dissipate. That doesn't seem to be the case, however. Why don't you get dressed and we'll talk."

She was alone again. She took off the johnny, slipped into her bra. Her hands shook as she hooked the catch behind her. Her hands shook worse as she buttoned her blouse. *So he couldn't aspirate it. He couldn't aspirate it. We're going to talk.* She went into Barry's office and sat. He was grim-faced. She was good at body language and she knew it was not good. He was grim.

"I know you're worried," he said. "That you are worried that this is an ovarian cyst. Ovarian? Oh God, I don't mean ovarian I mean mammarian cyst."

Joan said, "Jesus, Doctor, you're in worse shape than I am."

He laughed and his face went grim again. "The next step for you is a mammogram."

Joan said. "Okay." *Okay. Mammogram.* "I'm beginning to get scared of this, Doctor. Mammogram to me means I should start thinking about this as a malignant tumor."

"There's simply no way of knowing," he said. "Until we do further tests. The next test is a mammogram. You'll go over to Union Hospital and have a picture taken. A mammogram will give a much better idea. I think you should be thinking in terms of a biopsy, which is the only certain way to know what the lump is. And I would be happier if I could aspirate it. That's all I know now. And the next step is a mammogram."

She said, "Okay. If I need surgery, who would you recommend?"

He said, "Dr. Eliopoulos."

She nodded.

He said, "Are you going to be all right?"

She said, "Yup, I'm going to be all right. I haven't told my husband yet and I wonder if now is the time."

Barry said only what he could say. "It's up to you."

"I can't miss work," she said. "I can't miss work. I have to go on working." In three years she had not missed a class at Endicott College. She was puritanical about it.

"We'll schedule it in the afternoon," Barry said. "We'll try for tomorrow, but it's more likely to be Wednesday."

"But Wednesday my husband is speaking and I need to be there. I don't want to screw it up with a mammogram. He doesn't even know about this yet. And tomorrow afternoon I have to supervise a student who's taking over the classroom for the first time. It's important to her that I be there."

"And," Barry said, "we'll have to have the mammogram. We will tell the girl that we'll take the first appointment they have, and we'll work around that."

Joan said, "Okay. If this does lead to mastectomy how long will it be before I can work? What's the recovery time?"

"The surgery is not terrible. Say, ten days in the hospital. And most women are back on their feet in six weeks, four to six weeks."

They looked at each other for a moment, then Dr. Barry gave Joan's hand a small pat. "We'll hope for the best," he said. "And take one step at a time."

Chapter 4 ⌐

SHE DIDN'T drive straight home. She drove around town.
*There's no way now to say there's nothing to worry about. Barry
didn't come even close to saying this is nothing to worry about.
He hadn't said that this is not breast cancer. He didn't even come
close to saying that. I'm scared. I'm scared shit.* In the Center
on the common the white meetinghouse looked much as it must
have looked in the eighteenth century when it was built. The
spring night was silent and unoccupied around it. No cars, no
kids on the wall, no lights, except the empty arc of streetlights
on the aimless asphalt. She drove home and didn't tell Ace and
went to bed. *As long as he doesn't know and no one knows but
me I can pretend. When I'm with him or with others I can
pretend it's not true and all the people who are talking to me as
if it weren't true will make it seem as though it isn't so.* She
slept. Every few hours she woke and remembered and fell asleep.
During the waking periods she alternated between telling herself it wasn't cancer and beginning to deal with the possibility
that it was.

At four-thirty Tuesday morning she lay on her back in bed
and thought of Betty Ford and Happy Rockefeller. *All right.*

I remember them. It happened to them. And I remember saying to Jude and John that it all happened awfully fast. Betty Ford. Did they railroad her into a radical mastectomy because she was the President's wife and they didn't want to take chances with her life? Why didn't they give her an opportunity? Why wasn't there a chance to explore chemotherapy and radiology? Did some male chauvinist pig surgeon push her into a mastectomy because it was easier, safer for him, instead of trying the riskier newer approaches and thereby save the breast? I will not be railroaded. I am going to be very thorough and research this very well and, maybe, if it's breast cancer I can hang onto this breast. I will move on this slowly. And if it is cancer, say it is cancer, I will not be pushed. I'm not going to lose this breast because it's the quickest way, or the easiest for someone else. I'm not going to say, 'Yes Massah Doctor, whatever you say.' I'm going to make sure what I'm doing.

The dog, sleeping against the wall, half under one of the floor-length drapes as he always did, made a kind of lip-smacking sound and sighed and shifted his position. She got up. The bathroom door was ajar and the bathroom light was on. In the light from the bathroom she could see the dog now, lying on his side, the drape partially covering his head, his muzzle sticking out. He looked like Mammy Yokum. Ace on his side of the bed was motionless, his back to her, sleeping on his side. She went into the bathroom and looked at herself in the mirror. She took off her pajama top and looked at her breasts. She tried to flatten out the left breast by pressing down on it with her hand. *What does it look like? Grotesque. Gross. Unbelievable. A one-breasted woman. I can't believe it. Even flat, with boobs like mine you can't tell what it looks like and mine are easy to flatten. But you can't really tell.* They had paneled the bathroom in pine with a reddish stain and hung a big copper carriage lamp over the mirror. *Where does the incision go? Does it go up the shoulder? Down the back? Around the side? Under the armpit and around and meet the original scar? What do they do? Is it up? Down? Is it across? Christ, it's too awful. It's too much. I can't think about this. But I have to. I have to be prepared. If this happens to me I've got to be ready. Goddamn it, I will be ready. I will handle this.*

She put her pajama top back on and buttoned it. Her hands were steady. She went back to bed, stepping over the dog to do it and pulled up the covers and turned on her side and went back to sleep.

Tuesday, April 15

Work organized her morning. She taught her classes, focusing on the development of the young child and on the students, and handling it as well as she always did. She loved to teach, loved the students, and the sense of interacting lives that she found there. And the students gave it back. They were all girls and there was a sense of female community among them, teacher and student, of shared concern and shared awakening. Most of the administrators she thought suffered from near-terminal anality. But she loved the girls.

Her class ended at one-fifteen and she drove home and ate lunch, sitting on an antique blue stool at the chop-block counter in her kitchen. She had a half hour before she had to go and supervise the person whose take-over day it was.

The phone rang. "This is Dr. Barry's office. We have an appointment for your mammogram Wednesday at five P.M."

"Thank you very much." *So it will be Wednesday.*

Well, it's late, I'll be able to go to Ace's speech. She felt he needed her there. He usually needed her there. The speech didn't make him nervous, but he depended on her for the social bridge. His second novel was out, and he'd done some talk shows, but this was the big speech in the hometown at the women's club luncheon. Billy and Eileen, their oldest friends, were driving sixty miles for the luncheon and speech. Others were coming, Judy, June, Embeth. There would be a group back at the house afterward. She'd have time for that. Good. And at around five she'd excuse herself and go down to Union Hospital and get mammogramed and be back in a half hour or so.

"Days of Our Lives" broke for a commercial and she realized it was time for her to supervise.

Jean was an undergraduate at Tufts, majoring in Early Childhood Education and placed for her practice teaching at the Huckleberry Hill School, with Ruth Lenrow as head teacher and Joan as her supervisor. Today Jean took over the kindergarten, planning the activities and directing the children.

Joan concentrated on Jean's performance, on her relationship with the children, on her ability to redirect them, on her sense of the classroom dynamics. She sat quietly on a kid-sized chair and took notes. The children were used to her; she'd been there every week all term. There was a great deal happening in the classroom. It was relatively unstructured and the children moved from the doll corner and block corner to the math area and cooking projects in a boisterous tumble of movement and interest. It was late in the term. The children had gotten their place in the order of things worked out.

At snacktime Joan went into the other kindergarten to talk with Marcie Pitt, the teacher. Marcie was young, not long out of college, and Joan had helped her get the job. Joan had supervised student teachers in Marcie's classroom often and they had become friends. Standing beside Marcie at the sink, looking at the kids swirling earnestly about the open room, Joan said, "Marcie, I have a lump in my left breast."

"Oh, Joan," Marcie said, "what are you doing about it? What's happening?"

"I've been to the doctor and I'm having a mammogram tomorrow. No one is encouraging me to think it will be all right."

"Well they are always cautious," Marcie said. "My mother has had lumps and my aunt, and they were benign. Most of them are, you know."

"I know, but I'm scared shit, Marce."

"I know," Marcie said.

Why in hell, Joan thought. *Why in hell did I tell her? We're friends, but there are a lot of friends I'm closer to. Christ, I'm nearly twenty years older than she is, I could be her mother. Here we are in a classroom full of five-year-olds and I'm telling her something I've told no one else. What time could be a worse time? She hasn't got time for this.*

But the time and the relationship were about right. The situation structured the discussion so it could not last long, and could not get out of hand. Uncontrollable emotions couldn't well up and spill over. The work was there, and the children.

Marcie is a caring person, but it's not like telling Eileen, or Jude. Or Ace — Jesus, telling Ace. Marcie wouldn't care like they would, couldn't care like they would. It wouldn't devastate her. And Joan needed a woman to talk to. That was new for her. But now she needed someone female to bounce her emotions off of. She needed an outlet. She had told no one and now she had told Marcie. *Someone has to know how terrific I am.*

Joan saw herself, in part, as the central figure in a drama. And some of what she wanted from Marcie was audience feedback. She wanted Marcie to know that she was supervising and entertaining after tomorrow's speech and teaching her classes and conducting herself with grace under great pressure and burdening no one with her problem. She wanted Marcie to think, What A Fine Human Being. *What is the goddamn point of being terrific if no one knows you're being terrific?* Now someone knew. And tomorrow there was the mammogram, *tomorrow I'll be sure.*

Chapter 5 ⟶

THERE WASN'T a mammogram tomorrow. Tuesday night Norma Holloway, who worked in X-ray, called to say that the technician was sick and the appointment had to be canceled. Joan was frantic. Angry. Betrayed.

"You cannot cancel this, Norma. I can't have this canceled. I must have it." Norma was a neighbor. They had been friends for years. She felt her anger build, knowing as it built that it wasn't Norma's fault. She was just the messenger. And even in her desperation she was evasive. She still wanted her lump a secret. So she wouldn't speak of her lump. "I have been led to believe that a mammogram is imperative."

"Joan, what can I do? The technician won't be in."

Joan hung up and called Barry's office. She is close to tears. The closest so far. She is betrayed. *Gee, I'm really being a good kid. I'm doing it all. I'm keeping it to myself. I'm going through with the job and the speech and, goddamn, Norma calls me up and says it's canceled. Is the technician sick as I am? How sick can she be?*

She is teary on the phone with Barry's office. The secretary is kind and prompt. "I'm sure we can get you another appointment," she said. "Let me call and I'll call you right back." She did call right back. The appointment was Thursday; Joan would have the first appointment.

In a way it was good. Now Wednesday would be free and she could have her company and deal with Ace's speech and all without complication. One more day. *You could always do one more day. You could always get through one more day.*

Wednesday, April 16

They got the boys off to school. And were in the kitchen drinking coffee when she told him that her doctor appointment had been postponed. She'd warned him that she would have to go for another cauterization of her vaginal bleeding today, and now she said it would be tomorrow. "Nothing serious," she said.

He was leaning on the counter and she was sitting on one of the stools and he shook his head.

"What's going on?" he said. "There's too much hustling around to the doctor and too many little tests and too much oh-nothing-serious. What's wrong with you?"

She said, "Just some breakthrough bleeding, like I told you."

And he said, "No. There's something more. We've been together too long for me not to know something's up. Don't bull-shit me. It's always better to know than not to know."

Jesus, she thought, *he thinks I'm walking around with vaginal cancer. He's got the look. It's now. Speech or no speech. I'm going to have to tell him.* Later, looking back, she wondered why the speech had loomed so large. She felt so strongly that he should have serenity and stability before making it. Yet she realized now, it didn't mean that much to him. She just thought it did. Things had different proportions for her that spring. The opportunity to fulfill responsibilities seemed to be somehow a

stay against dissolution. For her to function, there had to be
something that mattered other than the lump in her breast.
Other things had to be important, so she could do them, otherwise the lump would consume her. But that she understood later. Then, in the kitchen, she knew only that the speech was
vital, but that she had to tell him.

And she said, "Listen, I'm going to level with you. I do have
a problem. It's a lump in the left breast and they have to x-ray
it to find out what it is. And I hope it's not malignant."

And he said, "The odds are pretty good, aren't they?"

And she said, "Yes. They are pretty good. My mother didn't
have breast cancer and neither did my sister or my aunts. It
doesn't run in the family and that makes the odds better. And
I'm not menopausal. That helps the odds."

He didn't seem too shaken. *In fact,* she thought, *he looks a
little relieved to know the truth.*

And he thought: *Lots of people survive breast surgery. Look
at Happy Rockefeller. Look at Betty Ford. If she's got it, it
doesn't mean she'll die.*

He said, "Everyone assumes if they have something it's the
worst. It's not that it's so likely, it's that it would be so terrible.
I do too. But that doesn't mean it is the worst. It's just as irra-
tional to assume it's cancer as to assume it isn't. All you have are
odds, and the odds are good." He knew he was saying the truth,
but the part of him that didn't care about knowing, that part felt
numb. *'Rose, thou art sick,'* he thought. *'The invisible worm
that flies in the night.'* But he hung on to the numbness. It
forestalled panic, and there was in him a consciousness of that
and a deliberate commitment to the numbness. At least for now.

She said, "I know that. I'm handling it. I'm all right."

And he patted her on the backside, as he did perhaps fifty
times a day. It was a gesture characteristic of their relationship,

equal parts camaraderie and love. She went to make the beds. He went to the package store for beer and wine. There would be people back after the speech and they'd drink.

The day organized them and carried them along. The speech at a local restaurant went well. The ladies were responsive, and the ham in him rose to their response. He enjoyed himself, getting laughter mixed with nervous ohhh's, as he made insulting remarks about his wife. "Life has no narrator," he said, "unless perhaps you're married to Joan Parker," and he looked over amid the laughter and saw her face bright and animated and thought about the lump. She was smoking, although she'd quit for more than a year. He knew why.

I can smoke a couple of cigarettes, she thought. *You're allowed a couple in this kind of trauma.*

"It comes at you random," he was saying, "haphazard. And the writer's job is to take the random happenstance and order."

It's good, she thought. *It's damn good. Am I sitting here listening to it with breast cancer? Is it possible I have cancer? Cancer. Cancer. Impossible. People with cancer are sick. Really sick.* She remembered her father who died of prostate cancer when she was nineteen. *The circles under the eyes, the dry heaves. The skin-and-bones body. That's what cancer is. Look at me. I'm Harriet Health for crissake. How can I have cancer?*

As she thought this she heard the speech and watched the ladies respond and felt good for him and was struck as she had been and as she would be so frequently that spring by the capacity to separate out the things that frightened her and the things that pleased her and to respond simultaneously to both.

The speech ended and they went back and sat in the sun-flooded family room and drank some beer and wine and had a good time. Later in the afternoon Joan and Eileen went shopping. Bill and Ace stayed with the beer.

As they shopped Joan went through the fantasy of telling Eileen. *My friend Eileen. I will say, 'Hey listen, Eileen, I have something to tell you. I have a lump in my breast'* . . . *Eileen is not ready to hear this. She has to shop. She's busy. What does she need from breast cancer? She'll have to dredge up the proper feelings and respond the proper way. She'll have to say, 'I'll help you through this. I'll stay by your side.'* They are in Marshall's and Eileen is trying on clothes. Joan looked in the mirror and thought, *maybe Jude, maybe I should tell her.* That was even more enticing. *Jude is a nurse. Maybe she knows something. Maybe she can tell by looking. Maybe she has a magic way.* Eileen comes out of the dressing room with a denim jacket.

"What do you think?" she said and turned slowly.

"Too big," Joan said. "It's nice but it's too big."

I can't tell Jude. I don't want John to know. I don't want any males to know. Especially I don't want any men to know. Don't think about it. Wait for the mammogram.

The Marshes came for dinner with the Ganems and it was ten-thirty before they were through cleaning up. Joan was exhausted. Ace lay on the living-room floor, talking to Daniel. The phone rang. Joan answered.

"Mrs. Parker, this is Sharon Taylor, in your Child Development Class?"

"Of course, Sharon. How are you?"

"Oh, Mrs. Parker, I've got a terrible problem."

Welcome to the club.

Chapter 6 ⌒

SHARON TAYLOR had to come and talk. "This is a terrible problem, Mrs. Parker. I can't talk on the phone. I have to come tonight to see you. You don't know what it's like. This is so awful." And Joan said, "All right, come over." And went down to tell her husband. *He'll be bullshit,* she thought. *He hates intrusions like this.*

"Don't get mad at me," she said. He was lying on the living-room floor, talking to the boys. "I've had a rough day and I'm exhausted. I'm begging you to let me do this without having a fit. I need to do this."

He knew why she needed to do this. "Yeah," he said. "Okay. I won't be mad at you." He thought. *Why the Christ can't she keep it separate? Why does she let the goddamned kids get at her? She's their teacher. She didn't hire on to be their goddamned mother.* "I'm betting pregnancy," he said. David at sixteen agreed. Dan at twelve thought it would be a school problem, and Joan agreed with Dan.

"The Dean's been mean to her," she said, "or she's been kicked out, something like that."

"Knocked up," Ace said.

"Pregnant," Dave said.

And they were right. Sharon Taylor arrived with four friends in a red-eyed flurry of anxiety and Joan took them upstairs to Dan's bedroom because it was more secluded.

Christ, here we are, sitting on the bed, we girls, smoking — I shouldn't be smoking — and talking about Sharon who's knocked up. It's like twenty years ago at Colby when we girls would sit on the bed in the dorm and smoke and talk about someone who was knocked up or thought she was.

Sharon wanted to abort the fetus. She had already decided that. In fact she had decided everything. She'd been to the pregnancy clinic; she'd made an appointment in Boston for an abortion Saturday morning. What she wanted from Joan was approval.

"We only did it once, Professor Parker. Just one time."

Shit luck, kid. You and me both, we have shit luck.

"You said in class that ovulation takes place twelve to fourteen days after the last period is over. But it didn't. We only did it once and it was just before my next period. You said it wasn't supposed to happen then."

"Don't get mad at me, hon. You either had a hell of a long-living egg or he had a hell of a viable sperm. Or you counted wrong. The point is, you're pregnant, whether you are supposed to be or not."

"Yes."

What is my function here? She's already decided to do the abortion. I'm supposed to give an adult okay. To tell her that she's still a good person even if she is pregnant. I'm supposed to say if I were she I'd abort. Well, I would.

"Have you talked with your mother?"

"Oh, God no, I couldn't tell her."

"Father?"

"They're divorced. I couldn't . . ." She shook her head. The other girls murmured and nodded. No one could tell one's mother or father.

"And Mike?"

"He wants to have the baby, get married right off and have the baby."

"You don't want that?"

"I love him, but I want to finish school. I don't want to get married yet. I don't want a baby. I want to keep going to school for another year."

Joan nodded. *This is grotesque, she thought. No, not grotesque . . . Ludicrous. Here I am up here at eleven-thirty at night smoking away — which I shouldn't, and the more I smoke the worse I feel — talking it over with the kids about pregnancy, and I'm walking around with breast cancer . . . Christ I'm almost ready to say it — breast cancer. I have said it. But I can't think about it. I have to think about Sharon and her pregnancy and how to make her feel okay about whatever she wants to do.*

"So," Joan said. "You're in a situation where there are no perfect solutions. But abortion seems the least imperfect to you." *Me and Carl Rogers. Restate for her.*

"I know, but we only did it one time." It was a litany. She wasn't old enough yet to accept imperfect solutions and problems that didn't solve, and she kept invoking her bad luck as if reminding the gods that her slip had been minor.

"But once was enough this time. It's down to a reasonably clear choice." Joan kept trying to refocus the discussion. The cigarette had gotten to her and she felt sick. For the first time since she discovered the lump she felt sick. *It's just the cigarettes. It's not the . . . lump. It's the smoking, it always makes everyone feel lousy when they're not used to it.* "You either marry Mike and have the baby, or don't marry Mike and have the baby, or you abort."

"But I don't want to marry Mike, yet."

"The baby won't wait."

"Oh, Professor Parker . . ."

It went on, mostly in a circle, until after one. Sharon left, committed to her abortion, and Joan stumbled into the bedroom exhausted. Dan was asleep on her side of the bed and she had to wake him and walk him, somnambulant, upstairs to his bedroom, which still reeked of cigarette smoke and anxiety. The exhaustion was valuable. She fell asleep at once and didn't wake until morning.

Thursday, April 17

Mammogram day. *What a sappy name for such an important occasion. Mammogram. Sounds like something you send on Mother's Day. Hello, Ma'am, here's your mammogram.* There was some tension in Ace's eyes, but not bad. *There's no Oh-my-God look there, she thought. He's okay.*

She went to Huckleberry Hill to supervise. He went to Northeastern to write.

Her supervision was a blur. She told Ruth Lenrow that she had a doctor appointment that afternoon.

"Is it anything big?"

"Ruth, it may be something really big. And I'm really scared about it."

"Oh, my God," Ruth said. "I hope it isn't bad."

"I hope it isn't, Ruth, but, Jesus, if it is bad, it's really bad."

What in hell am I doing? Why am I saying this? How can I say that and not tell her? It's worse than telling her the facts. But she didn't tell her, and Ruth's face showed the strain of compassion and uncertainty for the rest of the morning as Joan supervised.

As Ace checked his mail in the English Department, Ivy Derosier asked him if anything was the matter.

"How come no singing and whistling?"

"I'm thinking," he said. "It's very hard for me." It was a question he would hear and an answer he would give often that spring. It bothered him that it showed. If Ivy had noticed, how about Joan? *Grace under pressure,* he thought, as he rolled a blank sheet of paper into the typewriter. In the upper right-hand corner he typed Parker-Stakes-3. *Me and Santiago.* He had nowhere near her capacity for linear thought. His mind was always full of images and allusions. Pictures and scenes. But he was clearly aware of the surprise he felt that here in the crisis of his life he was thinking about Hemingway. *Sonova bitch* he thought. *Me and Santiago. Or Dilsey. They will endure. Faulkner and Hemingway and me. Amazing.* He concentrated on the story he was writing.

The last time Joan had been to Union Hospital was when Daniel had an emergency appendectomy. That was also the last time she had seen Gladys Carter — in the waiting room as they waited for the diagnosis on Dan and found he'd have to have emergency surgery. Last December.

When Joan walked into the waiting room at X-ray to wait for her mammogram, Gladys Carter was there.

Chapter 7 ~⌒

SHE HAD TO tell Gladys why she was getting x-rayed. Gladys promised to say nothing. From the beginning Joan's impulse had been secretive. Gladys would do what she said, but it was scary for her to be there again. *It means something bad is going to happen to me again.* Dan's surgery had always been something that had happened to her as much as to Dan. The nights sitting all night in a chair in the hospital, getting disapproving looks from some of the nurses, whose territoriality was impaired. The fear. *I'm headed for worse. Superstitious, very superstitious. But I am superstitious.* And yet it was good that Gladys was there. Gladys talked with her. It helped.

The mammogram technician was earthy and intelligent and informed and warm. The procedure was innocuous and painless. Wearing the inevitable johnny, Joan laid both breasts on a horizontal plate, between two perpendicular plates, and the pictures were taken from all sides. The technician took extra pictures of the left breast.

"When this is over with," Joan said, "will we know? Will somebody be able to say it is or is not malignant?"

"Yes. It's a wonderful diagnostic tool. You get a really clear idea of what you're dealing with."

"It will be good to know finally. Even if it's bad news, it will be good to be certain."

The technician nodded. "I know. Remember something like eighty-five percent of all lumps are nonmalignant. Your odds are very good."

In five minutes it was over. Painless, unembarrassing, easy. The results would be in tomorrow. Joan went home.

In the Cabot Gymnasium at Northeastern, Ace, in a gray T-shirt and white shorts, was lacing his sneakers. They were faded blue Adidas Varsities with one of the white stripes missing. *Working out when Joan maybe has cancer? Do what instead? I could go home and sit around and stare at her and say ohmigod a lot.*

He walked to the cage to the indoor track and began his daily twenty-two laps around it, two miles. He counted the laps by switching pebbles from one hand to another, and his mind was thus free to roam. That had always been useful to him in the past. He could work out plot complications, try out dialogue, imagine character as he ran. Today he thought about himself and Joan. As a concession to the steady low-grade ache in his stomach he'd had since she told him, he didn't run today against the clock as he usually did. Today he just did the twenty-two laps.

If she dies, I can make that. If she dies I will have the boys. I won't fold. I can do that. I can do whatever I have to do. I can do that. But, Jesus Christ, who will I talk to? Who will I screw? I'll want to. In a while I'll want to and who? I can't stand to do that dance again. Hi, my name's Bob Parker, what's yours? Do you have any hobbies? Shit!

It was a late spring afternoon and most of the runners were outside. The cage was nearly empty as he went around it, the sun shafting in through the high windows and silhouetting the particles of dust that always hung in the cage.

There's no point to this. Maybe she's fine. Maybe it'll turn out to be a sebaceous cyst. Thinking what if is no good. We'll take it as it comes and not look past it.

He finished the two miles and headed for the Universal trainer. He seemed to have no strength today. He couldn't bench-press what he had bench-pressed Tuesday. He had to force himself through the routine. *If she dies can I write, I wonder?* It was hard to imagine doing anything if she were gone. But the boys, he had the boys. *Funny, I don't think of them still having me. I think of me still having them.* He saw himself, his face a mask of controlled grief, with an arm around each of his sons. He snorted. *Bathos.* He pressed up the weight, exhaling hard as he did.

After supper, when they were alone in the kitchen, he said, "Do you want me home when you call Barry? Would you like me to call him for you?"

And she had said, "No, I think I better call him. I'll be okay."

He didn't pursue it. That spring they found that silence was a much better approach than talking, and that, oddly, staying apart was better than being together. There developed a kind of truce in their traditional commitment to discuss everything with each other. Talking made it worse, they realized, and sitting together in aching silence made the fear manifest. She went in the bedroom and lay down to watch television. He sat in the family room and read the *Globe*.

Friday, April 18

She went to work. The classes went well and after class she spoke to Judy Martin, the department head.

"Judy," she said. "I gotta tell you. I have a lump in my breast and yesterday I went for a mammogram. If the lump is malignant, and we'll hear today, you and I will have to figure out what to do with the rest of the term."

Judy Martin tried to be very upbeat. "Oh, Joan, don't worry about it. You know how often people have lumps and how it usually isn't bad."

"I hope so. Today we should know."

Driving home afterward Joan thought, *Jesus, now she knows. This is getting out of hand. Ace knows, and Marcie knows, and Gladys knows, and Norma knows, and Judy Martin knows, and who else? And for Christ sake there's probably not anything wrong with me.*

And on that warm April day, with the sun streaming into the car as she spun along Route 128, it didn't seem that anything was wrong. She had a new raincoat on, and she was driving the little hatchback Vega they had bought for her that was fun to drive compared to the station wagon they also drove. It was fun to drive because she felt in control of it. It was that feeling as she zipped along 128, looking good, feeling good, and in control that gave her a mystical sense of well-being. *I've got this under control. I do not have cancer. There's no way someone can feel as good as I do and be walking around with cancer. I'm not going to think about it. I'm not going to let it be cancer.*

That Friday he didn't go in. He was on sabbatical leave and went in only to write and use the gym. Today he didn't. Today he got the boys off to school and stayed home and walked around the house and looked at the clock. At one-thirty Dr. Barry's office would open and Joan would call and they'd know. After the boys had gone to school he stood a long time in the front door and looked out at the street, the same street he'd looked at for sixteen years. There was a stillness in him. And a need to breathe deeply from time to time. And tag lines and images from books he'd read and books he'd written flitted in the stillness.

It was ten o'clock in the morning. Three and a half hours. He could feel the burden of them pressing against his upper back. The trapezius muscles felt tense. He shrugged his shoulders. The dog was looking at him with the wise innocent face that dogs have, and he thought how he'd felt as a small boy when he had been punished and only the dog remained unchanged. There was no disapproval in dogs. But not all that much consolation either. They didn't know what the hell was going on. *Readiness is all.* He shrugged his shoulders again and walked through the house to the family room, and looked out at the woods, and the new growth that surged up as it did every spring. *'It is Margaret you mourn for.'* He thought about a bargain. *God, if the mammogram is okay I'll come back to the church.* He shook his head. *For crissake I can't do that. What kind of deity makes that kind of switch?* 'Okay, if you'll go to Mass every Sunday I won't kill your wife.'

"No," he said aloud. "No." *I don't want to do business with that kind of God. If he's there he'll do what he'll do, and if it involves trading faith for a tit I don't want him.* "If I do this," he said to the dog, "and Joan's okay I'll be superstitious all my life. I won't dare renege. If I do this and she's not all right I'll be ashamed." *And where does it end? Do I start making trades for a good review in the* Times? *For a movie contract? For a good reprint sale? If the kids have good checkups at the dentist I'll make a novena?* As he talked to himself he walked continuously. Back and forth from living room to family room, to bedroom to kitchen. The dog got used to the pattern and went to sleep on the living room rug, on his side, with his feet out straight.

Chapter 8 ⁓

AT ONE-TEN he called Dr. Barry. *Maybe he'll be there early. If it's bad I can be the one to tell her. If it's good she won't have to feel the tension of calling and waiting.* He dialed and waited while the phone rang. "Dr. Barry's office."

There was an eerie normalcy to it all. Just as if he were calling to find out what was playing at the movies.

"This is Robert Parker. Is the Doctor in?"

"I'm sorry, the Doctor won't be in until one-thirty. Is this an emergency?"

Oh, sweetheart, you don't know what an emergency this is. "No, thank you. I'll call back."

He called again at one-twenty, caught between the pressure of Joan's imminent arrival and the reluctance to call more than he had to. Barry was in.

"Hold the line, please," the secretary said.

As he held, Joan came in the door. "I've got Barry coming to the phone," he said. "Shall I talk or do you want to?"

"No," she said. "I better do this." Her palms were sweating and her stomach hurt as she took the receiver. He left the room and stood in the living room, where he could hear her but where she wouldn't have to watch him watching her. The stillness was in him. Joan could hear the office music as she waited. The voice on the phone said, "Dr. Barry."

"Hi, Dr. Barry, this is Joan Parker."

"Hi, Joan. We've got the mammogram results and you have a very, very, very suspicious mass in the left breast."

Three very's Joan thought. She said, "Uh-huh. Okay, what do we do now?"

"I want you to come in now," Dr. Barry said. "Do you have time?"

"Yes."

"It is time to talk with a surgeon about a biopsy."

Joan said, "Is it malignant?"

"There is only one certain way, Joan. That is a biopsy."

"I know, but would you guess? You probably don't want to guess, or give your feelings on whether or not it's malignant."

"Joan, the only way to know for sure is a biopsy. Do you have a surgeon you prefer or would you like to talk with Dr. Eliopoulos?"

"Dr. Eliopoulos is fine."

"Good. I saw him a half hour ago in the hospital dining room and we talked a little about you. He does not have office hours today, but he will come in to talk with you."

"When?"

"You should call him and arrange that. Tell him when it's best for you." He gave her the number.

"Okay." Joan didn't want to hang up. She wanted Barry to tell her something that would make her feel better. She wanted to say, "Can't you tell me something better?" But there was nothing to say. Nothing he could say. Joan said, "Okay, Okay. I'll call Dr. Eliopoulos," and she hung up.

She said to Ace, "It's a very, very, very suspicious mass, he said. I have to see Dr. Eliopoulos this afternoon."

"I'll come with you," he said.

"Yes."

"You want me to call?"

"No, I will."

"He couldn't say if it is certainly malignant?"

"No," she said. "He says a biopsy is the only certainty."

"That's what we'll go with then," he said. "So far we still don't know. And that's how we'll act."

The last vestige, she thought, *the last vestige of hope. Maybe the biopsy will come out negative. Very, very, very suspicious.* "Christ, that doesn't sound good," she said.

"What?"

"The very-very-very-suspicious. That doesn't sound good at all."

"No. It doesn't. But it sounds better than you-have-breast-cancer. We have to deal with what we have and not with what we fear. We know this much and that is what we know. We stay with what we know. We have to do that."

She nodded. "All the news is bad news," she said. "Never all week do we get any hopeful news. The whole week has been getting a little worse, and a little worse. I want to find out what the bottom is like." She dialed the number Barry had given her.

The secretary who answered knew Joan's name. Joan's voice was steady but it was very, very hard not to cry.

"The doctor will be here in a half an hour, and he'll meet you here in his office."

Joan said "Yah. I'd like to bring my husband."

And the secretary said, "Oh, my all means." *Very kind. Everyone is very kind. Oh God, this isn't good. They are too kind. They're really being too nice.*

They were kind, too, in the doctor's office. Joan and Ace were brought right in. Dr. Eliopoulos appeared at once. A tall man, with large strong-looking hands. Surgeony-looking Joan thought.

Joan lay on the table and Eliopoulos examined her breasts. The nurse stood by, and so did Ace, feeling oddly out of place and almost explosively protective. Joan could see him obliquely, leaning against the wall in the corner of the office, his arms folded across his chest, his face blank. It was a characteristic pose. *How often I've seen him like that.*

"Okay," Eliopoulos said. "When you get dressed, come in the office and we'll talk."

As Joan put her bra and blouse back on, alone with Ace in the examining room, both of them were thinking about being railroaded. *They're not railroading me,* Joan thought. *They're not pushing me into mutilating surgery because I'm a woman and it's easier for them than long-term management.*

She'll have what she wants, Ace thought. *It's her body and her life. I will see that she gets what she wants. But, Christ, I hope she goes for the surgery. I hope she doesn't fuck around with this and lose her life for a goddamned abstraction. I want this settled.* But she'd get what she wanted. He perceived his life in simple and somewhat dramatic terms. *That's what I'm for,* he often thought. *If they want something I see that they get it.* They didn't always get it, and he didn't always see to it that they did. He knew that too. But it was a guiding principle, and it helped him decide what to do.

In the office they sat across from Dr. Eliopoulos and he said, "Well, we'd better go ahead with the biopsy."

"And if it proves malignant?" Joan said.

"Then I feel we should go ahead and do a modified radical mastectomy."

"While she's still under?" Ace said.

"That's the best way. If it's malignant there's no point to two surgical procedures."

"Why a modified radical?"

"I don't do radicals," Eliopoulos said. "The survival rate, we've found is the same for modified radicals as it is for radicals."

"What's the difference?" Ace said. He didn't want to dominate a discussion that was hers more than it was his, but he knew how sick and numb she must feel and he plowed ahead. She'd interrupt as she wished.

"The so-called Halsted Radical," Eliopoulos said, "takes pectoral muscle as well as the breast. In the modified radical we don't take muscle."

"Why not just do the lump?"

Eliopoulos shook his head. He was never in doubt and the certainty with which he spoke and the fluency of his explanation had a part in their decision. He was very clear about what he thought. "A lumpectomy is not good medicine. I won't do it. There may be someone who will, but I can't. I think it's immoral. If you just excise the lump itself, you have absolutely no way to know if the malignancy has spread and if it has how far it has. This is an amorphous lump. It's outlines are not distinct."

"And chemotherapy," Joan said. Her voice was steady.

"Chemotherapy is a fallback position. If you start with chemotherapy and it doesn't work, then it's too late for the mastectomy and you have nowhere to go. Again. I won't do it. I think it's bad medical practice. There is one doctor in Boston who will do it, I think, and I can give you his name. But I can't do it."

"Why is it too late?" Ace said. *There's that harsh edge*, Joan thought. When he argued, or when he was after something, as he was here, he made her very uncomfortable. He had no skill to do it gracefully. When there was something at stake, a harsh rather ugly tone developed. He was capable of asking someone why six or eight times in a row, backing them down to the essence of their position. Usually she hated it. Here she did not. *We have to know*, she thought. *Go ahead, we have to know.*

Eliopoulos said, "As with the lumpectomy, you don't know what you're dealing with. You don't know how far it has spread and thus you are working blind. You need to biopsy the lymph nodes."

And it went on. Often over the same ground twice. Eliopoulos careful, thorough, unhurried, unoffended. After a half hour of very grueling discussion, Joan said, "We're taking too much of your time."

"No," Eliopoulos said. "No, that's perfectly all right. Take as much time as you need. It's an important decision."

"I don't mean to push you to the wall, Doctor," Ace said, "but I don't know how else to ask."

"I understand that," Eliopoulos said. "You have every right to get all the facts."

After an hour of question and cross-question Joan and Ace felt half disembodied, floating among the questions, in the clean medical room with the textbooks on the wall and the framed diplomas and certificates.

"I know what I think," Ace said. "But I won't tell you my decision till you've told me yours. It must be yours and I don't want to influence it."

Joan said, "Yes. I know what we'll do. On the operating table, if this lump has been removed and found malignant, a modified radical mastectomy is called for." She said it formally, carefully, as if saying it just right would help make the decision just right.

"I agree," Ace said. "That's what should be done. Do you wish to be awakened before they do the mastectomy?" He spoke to her as if Eliopoulos were not there.

"No, I see no point to that. Once it's started I'd like it done."

The decision was made and she never doubted it. For the sake of her life she was convinced it was right. And she had another turn down the spiral. Now she was no longer thinking about saving the breast. Now she was thinking about living or dying. She was where he had begun. He had never cared about the breast, except that she had. He had always worried about life or death.

"Okay," Eliopoulos said. "I'd like to have you come in Sunday, Sunday afternoon. Check-in time at Union Hospital is three o'clock, I believe."

"Can I have a private room?"

"We'll try for that."

"Oh, Doctor," Joan said, "I beg of you that I have a private room."

"We'll try. I'll tell them it's important. Even if you don't get it the first day, I'm sure we can get one soon."

"Price is irrelevent," Ace said, and felt like a fool saying it. *So corny, so typical, so middle-class, middle-aged, overweight paterfamilias. The best money can buy. Spare no expense, my good man.*

"Monday and Tuesday we'll do some tests," Eliopoulos said. "Bone scans, body scans, that sort of thing. Nothing unpleasant, and Wednesday morning we'll do the biopsy."

They both nodded. They didn't ask about the scans. They knew he meant x-ray scans and they knew it was to see if the cancer had spread. They were a long way down the spiral now. Now they were willing to settle for a breast. *A simple boob, for crissake.* Now they were hoping it was only breast cancer and that it was not infesting her body. Now they were praying for only mastectomy. Each step along the process caused more anxiety. Each diagnosis presented worse possibilities. It was a week now since she'd found the lump. A week of excruciating anxiety. The anxiety and the uncertainty were exhausting. And the jagged descent of her hopes, and the effort to control them left her almost disoriented. Last Friday night she'd found the lump and gone to sleep and Saturday it had not disappeared. Monday she'd gone to Barry's office and he had not said, "Oh, it's just a benign cyst." Thursday the postponed mammogram had not dispelled her fears. Today her talk with Eliopoulos had confronted her with the possibility of metastasis.

For Ace the descent had lasted only three days, but he had begun farther down the spiral and his mind had never been preoccupied with worries about losing a breast. He felt a little lightheaded as they walked out of the office and into the bright spring day. The fear was a palpable weight in his chest, dragging downward on his shoulders, causing him to slump. He caught himself, and straightened. *Two more days and she goes in the hospital. I want this over,* he thought. *I want somewhere along the line to know something.*

They didn't speak of it, as during that spring they spoke of very little, but they both at one level of consciousness speculated on how much the need to end the uncertainty influenced their decision. To have gone to another doctor and gotten a second opinion, or to have agreed only to a lumpectomy and then found a doctor to do chemotherapy, would have postponed certainty, perhaps for months. *We had to know,* she thought. *We couldn't have stood that,* he thought. *Am I giving up a breast just because I can't stand the uncertainty?* she thought. *Did I let her go this route too easily because I don't have the strength to hold out and exhaust all other avenues?* he thought.

Their fear was of what they didn't know. It was a fear of what they might have to undergo, a fear that she might suffer, a fear that she'd be disfigured, a fear that the mastectomy wouldn't work and the cancer would spread and there would be other operations and other uncertainties. There was fear that she would linger in pain and there was fear that she would die. The fear was very large and varied. Like a conglomerate rock, and binding the conglomerate was the other fear. The fear that they couldn't handle it. That one would let the other down, that they would both let the children down. The fear that when they met the beast in the jungle, they would fail.

What will I say to her? he thought.

"Ace, I can't stand this," she said. Her face was red and tight.

"Yes, you can," he said. "We'll do this. We'll take it a step at a time." *What can I say to her? How can I get us through this? What if she can't do it?* It was very hard to be tough. So much harder to be tough when you really needed to be. When there was something to be tough about. It was much harder to be tough than a lot of people who spoke of it ever had a chance to know.

The feminists. She thought. *When you read about this kind of thing and hear people talk about how the sexist pig doctors want to snip off your boob . . . all that sounds so good. The sexist bastards will never get me. But then when you have a malignant breast and you might die if they don't remove it and there's just you and Ace to decide and you feel like you might die from the awfulness of it before the cancer can even get you, and you're terrified, then it doesn't sound as simple as they made it.*

"Did we do the right thing?" she said.

"Yes," he did.

"Eliopoulos is right, isn't he? He's not just railroading us. You're convinced, aren't you?"

"Absolutely," he said.

"The feminists . . ." she said.

"Fuck them," he said.

Chapter 9 ⟿

THE DENIAL URGE was strong in her as they drove away from the Medical Building. *Wednesday I'm having surgery and they will probably take my breast. I can't believe it. I cannot believe it.*

"Listen," Joan said, "I don't have a thing to wear." It was a typical remark of hers, no matter where she was going. He almost smiled. "We've got to go to Marshall's," she said. He turned up Route 1 and headed for the discount store. "We've got to get a nightgown and slippers," she said.

As they walked through the aisles at Marshall's, Ace pushing the carriage, she was thinking, thinking. *Gotta get a robe. If they do it, I've gotta get a robe that will obscure the imbalance as best it can.* "I don't want a see-through jobby," she said. "I don't want anything sexy."

"It's gotta be more sexy than the sweat pants and surplus fatigue jacket you have been wearing," he said.

"It's gotta be kind of a utilitarian robe, that could easily be padded out when they do it." She didn't say "if," and he didn't correct her. Neither had any real doubts, just a very small hope, up there in the corner, almost out of sight.

Marshall's was a clothing store that sold seconds, samples, and such from bins along the aisles, and had pipe racks everywhere. He hated it there. She loved it. He felt the same itchy boredom he always felt when he shopped with her, a boredom always slightly modified by the pleasure of being, however unromantically, alone with her, out of the ordinary context of home and yard.

He was aware of the garish normalcy of the way he felt, juxtaposed with the desperate purpose of their shopping. 'The torturer's horse scratches his innocent behind on a tree,' he thought. 'About suffering they were never wrong, the old masters.' Christ, now I'm quoting Auden.

Joan's concentration on the choice of a robe represented a kind of lifesaving struggle to proceed normally in the face of a mortal possibility.

"What to wear to a mastectomy," she said to Ace. They were at the robe rack. "That's no good," she said. "That one would gap. And that one is too filmy. People coming to see me don't want their attention called to my chest." He nodded.

"Makes sense," he said.

She picked out two robes. "These lend themselves to the one-breasted bod," she said, "rather nicely."

"Chic," he said. "Chic as a bastard."

She bought two padded bras. *If the breast goes I can wear the padded bra and shove something in it and maybe it will look okay.* She talked to herself almost without interruption, a lively, animated, and entirely consuming dialogue. *You know, I can receive visitors, and I can look all right.* She knew that later, after the hospital, she would be fitted for a prosthesis. She had always hated the word. Her concern was for the first few days after surgery, before the imbalance could be modified, when the first visitors came.

And so she planned. She bought slippers and a nightgown.

And she felt a little better. It was like planning for a trip they had to take although they weren't that keen on going. She was that way. She never allowed things to happen. She planned for them. She had to have an impact on the events. She could not stand randomness. It was a form of control. If you planned enough and thought about things enough they did not slip up on you and start running around loose. If you concentrated on them you could get hold of them. And she needed all her life not to have things run loose. She needed a hold.

And so she planned. *Now I have things to wear to the hospital. All right, the next thing is to tell the boys. We will go home and I will tell the boys that I am going to the hospital.*

"How much do we tell them?" she said, when they were back in the car.

"They shouldn't have to carry what we're carrying. But they have a right not to be bullshitted."

She nodded. "We'll tell them I'm having a cyst removed."

"Yeah. That's fair. That's the truth as far as we know it. We don't have to speculate for them, or lead them into speculation of their own."

"And if they ask about mastectomies and cancer? Betty Ford's been in the news."

"We'll say it's nothing to worry about."

"That's bullshitting them."

"Yeah, it is, but only a little and they shouldn't have to be where we are. Not yet. If it happens it happens and we'll tell them. But if it turned out to be just a cyst, they'd have been worried for nothing."

"That's not likely," she said.

"I know," he said. "But it's possible."

She was thinking, *They'll be revolted at the idea of me with one breast.*

He was thinking, *They'll be worried that she's going to die.*

"I guess we can lie to them a little," he said. "When they were small we lied to them about Santa Claus and the Easter Bunny. I don't see why we can't lie to them a little here. At least until we know."

She nodded. "Until we know. There's no need for them to deal with the not-knowing. We'll tell them the truth when we have a truth to tell them. And we'll do it all along the way. We'll tell them what we know."

It was late afternoon as they pulled into the driveway. Dan met them at the door.

"Where have you been?" he asked, the annoyance showing in his voice.

"We've been to the doctor's," Ace said, annoyed at Dan for being annoyed.

"And we had to do a little shopping," Joan said. "Come on in and I'll tell you about it while Daddy gets supper."

David was sitting at the table in the family room drawing. Joan and Daniel sat on the couch, while Ace made chicken breast in white wine, and rice pilaf for supper.

"Sunday I'm going to have to go to the hospital for a couple of days," Joan said, "and have a cyst taken out of my left breast."

"Is it anything serious?" David asked.

"It's a cyst," Ace said from the kitchen. "Remember when I had one removed from my neck?"

"It's nothing to worry about," Joan said. "I'll be in the hospital a few days."

"Can we come and visit you?" Dan asked .

"Yes," Joan said. "Daddy will bring you down."

"Will you be in the same part I was?" Dan asked.

"Daniel, you were in the pediatric ward," David said. "She's not a kid."

"All right, I was just asking."

"Well, it's pretty dumb to think she's going to be in the pediatric ward."

"Shut up, shut up, David. Just shut up."

I guess they're not too worried, Joan thought. *But I mustn't forget what I know about kids. Things like this take a while to sink in. They won't assimilate it right away. But later there may be some fallout.*

"You're such a baby," David said.

"I wasn't talking to you anyway. Why don't you just shut up," Dan asked.

Ace exploded from the kitchen. "Both of you shut up, goddamnnit."

Joan got up and went toward the bedroom. "I'm going to lie down for a while," she said.

At seven-fifteen that evening she called Judy Martin, at home.

"I'm sorry," she said, "to call you at home, Judy, but I've been having tests, as you know, and the mass is quite suspicious. I'm having a biopsy on Wednesday and then we'll know for sure. But I think it's time we talked about the rest of the year."

"Oh, Joan, I don't think you should be worrying about that now."

"No, I should. Dr. Barry said that if it's malignant the recovery period would be four to six weeks. That means I won't be back this term."

"I'm sure . . ."

"Now here's my plan." Joan plowed ahead. It was important to get it all said just right, and to get it all said, and to forestall the need for awkward expressions of sympathy. Judy Martin had never been especially articulate and Joan wanted now to get past her empathy. "I can tape a whole bunch of lectures ahead of time, and Ace can bring them in and play them. He's on sabbatical and he can be the teacher, playing the tapes and answering questions. It will be a kind of continuity. Then after surgery we can assess where we are."

"My God," Judy Martin said, "will he do that?"

"Yes."

"Well, I hope he doesn't have to."

"I hope so too, Judy. But I'm pretty sure that I won't be back this term." *Or maybe ever.* The phrase popped up in her head and she pushed it back down. *Too busy. Too busy to think about that. Too much to do.*

"Anything I can do," Judy Martin said.

"I know, thank you. I'm going in Sunday, so Big Bobbo will be in Monday with the tapes. And then every Monday, Wednesday, and Friday."

There was a moment of uncomfortable silence. Judy Martin was having some surgery soon on an injured leg and they both felt some empathy. But there was nothing else to say.

When Joan hung up she felt the panic beginning to rise. She had so much to do. All that taping, and the house. *Jesus, the house. What if I don't come home? I don't want anyone to see the house messy.* She had a picture in her head of the mourners coming back after the funeral to sit in the living room amidst the disarray that she had left. *Ace will never get it clean. He thinks he does, but he doesn't see like I do. He thinks it's clean when he does it, but it isn't. 'Poor Joan,' they would say, 'it's not like her to have left her home like this.'* So she began to clean. As she cleaned she thought of all the taping she had to do, and of the parade. She'd have to go to that goddamned parade tomorrow, and yet there was so much to do. *And then I'll have to tape all those lectures, and I've only got tomorrow afternoon and Sunday morning. And the house is a mess. Christ! Why doesn't someone help me?*

It got worse. Sharon and Mike came and sat in the family

room with them and talked of tomorrow's abortion. Mike especially acted on the premise that no one had ever loved as he had.

I remember that, Ace thought. *Hell, I still feel that way.*

They talked of Mike's upcoming Air Force enlistment and Sharon's last year of school. Of the year they'd be apart.

"You don't know what it's like," Mike said. "To face this kind of separation."

Ace and Joan looked at each other without expression. *Jesus Christ,* Ace thought, *this is incredible. I may kill them both.* But both of them knew that Mike and Sharon's story threaded into their own was a great plus. It was another something to think about.

"I did miss Joan when I was in Korea," Ace said, "but it's probably not the same."

Chapter 10 ~

Saturday, April 19

THE BICENTENNIAL Patriot's Day. Concord and Lexington and Jerry Ford coming to call and a mass of tourists. It was the kind of event Joan never went to. It was the kind of event that Ace went to with the boys and she stayed home. Eight days ago she was not planning on this one either. But the fear was growing that they were not talking merely about her breast, that perhaps they were talking about her life. *Is it possible*, she thought, *is it possible that my days are numbered* . . . The quaint phrase, out of a nineteenth-century melodrama, seemed so inappropriate to the reality she faced. And yet it was the phrase that had popped into her head.

It's something I should do. The family together, the nation's birthday. There was a vague sense of heritage and tradition as a stay against impending dissolution that propelled her. It would make a good memory. *It will also reassure the kids. How sick can Mamma be if she goes to the parade with us? They didn't seem worried, but they would be at some point and this would help.*

The big events were in Concord, but Ace said it would be too crowded and they went instead to Boston for the parade and festivities at City Hall Plaza. Had Joan been well he might have made a stab at Concord and Lexington, but he couldn't say that and merely insisted that it would be too crowded.

The crowds were not a problem in Boston. They parked near the Old State House and walked up across City Hall Plaza and over Beacon Hill to Boylston Street. It was a good day in April. Sunny and filled with a sense of festival. Street vendors sold balloons, and hot dogs, and frozen yogurt on a stick, and macro-biotic rice and lentils, and Granny Smith apples, and toy colonial sabers, and three-cornered hats. It was not yet nine o'clock and the city was pleasant and uncluttered, the way it is early on a nonworking day.

Joan had on her new raincoat, light poplin, and stylishly cut. She walked, *like Napoleon,* she thought, with her hand inside her coat, feeling the lump unconsciously over and over, always hoping futilely and below the ordinary level of her consciousness that if she felt it enough it would go away.

Ace loved the city. When he was working at home he would often invent an excuse to go in and drive around. He needed contact with it, and was always persuaded that if he lost contact with it his creativity would dwindle. *Is that hokey? That's the kind of crap they say at suburban poetry clubs. Erich Segal would probably say that. Or Rod McKuen. Arf!* But he felt it, and he felt it now.

He knew why she was here. She hadn't said and neither had he, but he knew. And it pleased him. He always wanted her to come along when he went places and he always wanted to go places. She did not enjoy going to places and she didn't enjoy traveling. *Sort of extreme provocation,* he thought, *but you take what you can get.*

He considered whether he ought to be guilty about being glad she'd come, even though what caused her to come was dreadful.

He decided he ought not to feel guilty. *We better take what we can out of whatever comes our way. And we better feel what we can feel and not fuck it up with worrying about whether what we feel is right.*

He was more at home with randomness than she was. He planned what he could: trips, building projects, that sort of thing. He outlined the novels carefully. But he knew the world to be essentially haphazard and he tried hard to take it as it came. And he knew that he was imperfect and would fail often and that, too, he would have to live with.

So he felt glad about her being along and paid attention to the parade. It came in a flourish of pennants and batons and braid and Ancient and Honorable Artillery companies. There were militia companies from around the Commonwealth, and drum and bugle corps in bright sateen costumes, led by plump-legged majorettes in white boots. There was a good deal of humor at the expense of the plump-legged majorettes.

"Look at this one," Dave said, as a particularly sturdy set of cheerleaders led a high school band past them.

"Look at the one in the middle." Dan shrieked with laughter.

"I think the band motto may be Bow Wow," Ace said.

"Sexist bastards," Joan said.

"It's Phil Spitalny and his all-hound orchestra," Ace said.

After the parade had passed they walked up Boylston Street and ate lunch in Ken's restaurant. Their table was on a second-floor balcony that looked out over the plaza in Copley Square. The fountain was working and the rush of its waters patterned the plaza and modified Boylston Street. Things quickened about it.

It's like being glazed over, Ace thought. *It's like having a thick layer of polyurethane varnish which seals you off from the elements. The fountain and the plaza are beautiful and the lunch is good and the family's together and my wife has a cancer growing. And we go along on two simultaneous levels and feel both things and they don't seem to connect. The two levels. They just seem to coexist laminated, separated by an invisible shield. Emotional Gardol.*

Walking back to the car after lunch, across the Common, they saw fragments of the parade now over, groups of bandsmen and majorettes, and sections of bugle corps and muster companies wandering at easy random back toward buses and cars that would take them home. Church bells rang periodically around the city. Family groups were frequent. The sun shone. The temperature was mild. In City Hall Plaza in front of the magnificent Stonehenge of the new City Hall there were thousands sitting on steps and standing on the bricked piazza waiting for Arthur Fiedler to conduct the Pops, and for a horde of pigeons to be released, and for the first of many speeches. The vendors were among them. Joan and Ace and the boys waited and watched for a while, but no pigeons appeared and Arthur Fiedler wasn't leading the Pops and Ace could see the tightness in Joan's face. Over some objections from the boys, they finally left in midafternoon and drove home.

She was alone in the house that Saturday afternoon. Her husband and her sons were out together. She knew the absence was contrived. Ace felt she needed to be alone. The strain was greater in front of the boys, not looking worried, not seeming down, not being snappish. Now there was less strain. But the panic moved in, as if to replace the strain. *Nature hates a vacuum.* She was busy, very busy: her notes, her tapes, her cleaning. And always the panic, seeming always to be intensifying, thrust back, pushed down yet growing, growing.

She was plugging in the vacuum cleaner when Norma came across the street and stuck her head in the front door.

She said, "Joan?" and her face had a look of great sadness. "How are you doing, Joan?"

Joan began to cry. "Norma, oh God, Norma I'm so scared."

"I know, honey. I know, I know." She put her arms around Joan and patted her and Joan cried against her as she hadn't since she'd found the lump.

They sat on the couch in the living room. "I'm sorry," Joan said. "I'm sorry I'm crying, but I'm so scared."

"I knew from the mammogram," Norma said. "I knew you'd be upset."

"Norma, what the hell is happening to me?"

"What's the next step?" Norma said. "What happens now?"

"I go in tomorrow and they do some tests. Wednesday they do a biopsy and if it's bad they do a mastectomy right then."

Norma nodded. Joan had the crying under control now. She could talk. "But I need to know what it means, Norma. I need to know what the hell it's like, what really happens, you know?" I mean they are all nice as hell. Eliopoulos, Barry, everybody, but what's it going to be like? How bad will it hurt? What's it like without one? Will I be all right? Jesus, Norma, it's so scary."

"I'll put you in touch with a woman I know," Norma said. "She had it done about a year and half ago."

"Who?"

"Gretchen Benjamin. She would be terrific for you to talk with, because she took it really well. Like nothing. It really didn't seem to bother her that much."

"Oh, Norma. My God, where did she get the courage?"

"She may have been putting on a wonderful show, but it didn't seem to bother her. And she made a good recovery."

"Is she all right now?" Joan said.

"Fine. She's a little tired sometimes, but otherwise she's doing fine," Norma said.

A little tired. That's not bad. They say Betty Ford's a little tired. If I have to feel a little tired that won't be so bad. Gretchen Benjamin actually had a mastectomy and survived and is walking around leading a normal life.

"How long did you say it was?" Joan asked.

"About a year and a half ago," Norma said. "And then later, of course, she had a hysterectomy."

Joan said, "What do you mean? She had a hysterectomy as a result of her mastectomy?"

"Well, yes, in a sense," Norma said. "They do that quite routinely. It's the hormones. They don't want the ovaries pumping out hormones, so they have to remove the ovaries. It's quite common."

Joan began to cry again. "Oh, my God, Norma. I don't want a hysterectomy."

For reasons she never understood, abdominal surgery had always seemed particularly fearsome. Dan's appendectomy had frightened her badly. But it was more than the terror of abdominal surgery. *My God, am I going to have a mastectomy, then a hysterectomy? What are they going to do to me? Are they going to chop away at my body? Is there cancer everywhere? I don't want to live by being chopped into little pieces. One year we'll take this, and another year we'll take that.*

But in the middle of the despair was the inevitable counterpoise. Gretchen Benjamin had handled it well. *If she can, I can.* She could feel the competitive flush in her. *She can't be a better person than I am. How come I'm not handling it well?*

"Have you told Judy yet?" Norma said.

"Jude? I can't tell Jude. I didn't want to tell you, Norma. I don't want anybody to know what happened to me."

"Oh, Joan, you're insane." Norma said. "Judy would be the perfect person to tell. She's your close friend. She's a nurse. She works at the hospital you're going to be in. She can special you on the surgery day. Wouldn't you like to have Judy Marsh there when you wake up. Wouldn't you want to talk to her?"

"Of course," Joan said. "But I don't want to burden anyone else with this knowledge. If I survive this I don't want anyone to perceive me as deformed. To walk into the room and see me and think 'There's One-Tit Tillie over there. Now which side was it? Which one is the fake?' Norma, do you know how much of our humor is involved in boobs? I mean, Christ, it is a subject that comes up all the time. I don't want people walking around saying, 'We better not use boob humor, we better get off the subject of boobs.' I don't want people starting to joke and then smothering it and trying to cover it up by misdirection because it might make me uncomfortable. We are a boob society and everybody will have to watch their mouths because of me and cancer, and, you know, I'll be a drag to have around."

Norma was shaking her head. Joan plunged on. Elaborating an argument she'd had with Ace. "If nobody knows then nobody will have to feel that way. They can feel the same way about me. If nobody knows they don't have to worry and I don't have to worry. Gretchen's walking around and no one would know, right, Norma? I mean she's got full use of her arms?"

Norma said, "No, of course you wouldn't know to look at her."

And Joan said, "That's it. That's what I mean. Nobody is going to know. That's the way I want it. Particularly the men. John Marsh, or Billy Ganem. I don't want them to know. I don't want them to perceive me as any less of a sexy person. Assuming they think I'm sexy now. I can't bear to have people sorry for me, to limit their conversation when I'm in the room. And I can't bear to be the kind of person that when they see me reminds them of cancer and dying. I can't do it."

Norma nodded. "Sure. I understand that, but look at it from this point of view. If you don't tell Judy she's going to find out.

You're going to Union Hospital. She works in Union Hospital every other weekend. There's no way that she won't find out. It's inconceivable. One way or another she'll know, and why not tell her now so she can help you?"

"Why does she have to know?" Joan said. "She's not working this weekend, and maybe next weekend I'll be home."

"What about Grace down the street? Grace works in the operating room. What if Grace says to Judy, 'How's Joan recovering from her surgery?' And Judy didn't know. How will she feel?"

Joan said, "She'll feel bad."

Norma said, "That's right. She'll feel excluded, or whatever, that you haven't told her, of all people. This is a very meaningful piece of information. Sharing it with her is a testimony to your friendship."

"Maybe, Norma, maybe you're right. I just don't know. But I will think about it."

Norma left to call Gretchen Benjamin and have her get in touch.

Joan walked around the house, crying again. Now that she had begun it was easier. She hadn't cried before. *Now I'm making up for it,* she thought. Across the street was Judy's house. As it had been for ten years. *She's in there and I've got to tell her.*

Chapter 11 ~

SHE WALKED across the street and into the Marshes' weathered-shingle Cape and said, "Jude, I need to talk with you alone."

Judy sent the kids to another room looking befuddled. In ten years Joan had never said, "I must speak to you alone."

I wonder if she knows, Joan thought. *She worked last night. I wonder if she knows, and is having the good taste not to mention it until I do.*

"Jude," she said, "do you know what's wrong with me?"

"No. Is something wrong with you?"

"A week ago — " *My God, only a week ago* — "I discovered a lump in my left breast and, Jude, they tell me it is malignant, that it's cancer and I'm walking around with breast cancer." As she spoke she began to cry again. Judy didn't cry. She held together. *She's not a crier.* Joan thought. *I don't usually cry in front of people. She doesn't cry, period.* But her face seemed to pinch in and get smaller. She was very fair with blond hair and blue eyes. As Joan talked her skin got paler and the eyes seemed to occupy more and more of her face. But she didn't cry."

What a terrible thing to do to her day, Joan thought in the uninvolved corner of her brain, which had been calmly observing the rest of her since the lump appeared. *But I don't care. I have to tell her, I have to let down with someone.*

Judy didn't assimilate it all at once. "You had the mammogram?"

"Yes."

"But, Joan, you always too such good care of yourself. You have tests done regularly."

"I know, Jude, I know."

"And you've been examining your breasts?"

"Yes, but since the first of the year, for the last three months or so, I haven't been doing it as carefully, and, my God, Jude, this thing is huge, where the hell did it come from? It's like a walnut."

"And you've had the mammogram?"

"Yes."

"Joan, we just have to think it's going to be okay. Even if you have the mastectomy, we just have to assume it's going to be okay."

Joan was beyond worrying about the mastectomy, and didn't try to pretend with Judy. Joan was worried about dying. "If this is in the rest of my bod, Jude, and we have to go through a series of operations to stop the onslaught . . ."

"It won't be that way, Joan. Don't think about that. It will be all right. It hasn't had a long time to grow. It hasn't had a long time to spread. You have regular checkups. It's going to be all right. It's going to be in time."

"Norma suggested that you might special me, Jude."

"Of course."

"Do you think it will be all right to have you special me?"

"Why wouldn't it be all right?"

"Well," Joan said, "it might be embarrassing. What if I were a terrible patient, Jude? What if I were yelling and screaming and out of my head? Or if I'm mean and horrible? I wouldn't want you to see me that way."

"Oh, God, Joan, you're not going to be like that. You'll be fine. I'll be right there. I can give you your medication as soon as you need it. People are okay after surgery; there's no screaming and yelling."

"I've never had surgery, I don't know what I'll be like."

"You'll be like you are," Jude said. "Like you were after the babies."

Joan was well past worrying now if she'd lose her breast. She was worrying about postoperative behavior. "Will I be a good patient?" she asked. "Will I be out of my head? Will I be ashamed of myself? What does the anesthesia do to you? Do you get cuckoo? Are you in extreme pain?"

"There's medication," Judy said, "to carry you after surgery. There's no screaming and yelling. You don't get crazy. I'll be right there."

I can't believe Jude and I are having this discussion, Joan thought. *Sitting here in her living room and talking about recovery from cancer surgery. God, it's hard.* But harrowing though it was it was also a release. Joan was glad to have gotten it done, and to know that Judy knew and that when the time came Judy would be with her. She needed the support of a woman. Since her trial had begun she'd found to her surprise that she needed the support and care of other women. She'd always been a man's woman. She'd preferred the company of men, found them more interesting, found most women duller than the men. As she had moved into a career in her middle thirties, returning to school for graduate work, and going on to become a professor, she'd found women more interesting, and as the feminist movement had progressed she'd realized more and more that some of her preference for men was an assumption of their superiority. Her tastes had been changing over the last five or six years. But never before had she sensed the need for women that she had now. Other women knew. Men, even Ace, didn't know.

"Don't tell John," she said.

"Joan, I . . ."

"I don't mean ever. I know you have to tell him. But not tonight. Not until we've been to dinner and come home and you and he are alone. Just that. Just this one thing. Okay?"

And Judy said, "Of course."

"It's just that it's the last night out for a while and I don't want it spoiled with thoughts of death and cancer hanging in the air. You and I and Ace can pretend. And John doesn't have to deal with it till tomorrow."

It was probably more than that. There was still the sense that men would think of her as maimed. That once John knew, he would no longer be able to think of her in sexual terms. He could no longer find her desirable. He could no longer imagine that she might be fun to sleep with. She sensed that very strongly, and she never swerved in her conviction that the men who knew could never again look at her with desire. Except Ace. She knew with even more certainty that he would feel exactly the same about her. She never doubted that he would desire her with the intensity that he always had. She knew it would never matter to him. But to everyone else, she knew it would.

And so for one final evening she wanted to still be sexy. She wanted to be whole and desirable and unscarred in John's imagination. Of these feelings she was inarticulately aware. They were less an idea than a sensation at the time. But she knew that one more time she didn't want John to know. One more evening.

Chapter 12 〜

SHE TRIED to explain to Ace later why she didn't want John to know. He was shaving, she was dressing.

"If we all know," she said. "The evening will be awful. But if three of us are keeping it from the fourth it will give us a chance to have fun and a way of dealing with the gloom. You know?"

"Yep." He leaned in closer to the mirror and stretched his upper lip down to get the whiskers on his upper lip, close to his nose. "I go along with that."

"John can still think of me as sexy, or attractive, or whatever. You know?"

"You don't have to worry about that, my love." He ran the tips of two fingers over the shaved area under his nose. "He thinks you're a hound anyway."

"Well, just once more he can think of me as a two-boob hound anyway. Okay?"

"Okay."

The Hilltop Steak House was an enormous milling flamboyantly middle-American restaurant, which served excellent food. The various dining rooms in the Hilltop were named after western cow towns and seating was by the deli-counter numbers method. A loudspeaker ran during the entire dinner: "Number three sixty-seven for Kansas City...Number eighty-one for Dodge City." The Hilltop served large quantities at low prices. It was crowded with fat people in stretch fabrics, managed and controlled by several tough-looking Saugus cops, all of which offered the Marshes and the Parkers frequent opportunity to say something funny. And they always ate and laughed in a kind of camp good humor at the unstylishness of it all.

"Nice outfit," John murmured, as they sat in a booth. A short fat man came in with a tall woman who wore a lot of rouge and had artificially blond hair teased high in a bee's nest. He was wearing red-checkered pants and white shiny loafers with a matching white shiny belt, and a trendy-looking maroon Qiana body shirt unbuttoned halfway to his navel. His hair was modishly cut and heavily sprayed and he had beads, worn tight around his neck. A thick roll of fat wallowed out over his belt.

"It's a look I've been trying to achieve," Ace said.

Judy said, "Oh, my God, look at her."

The blond woman had enormous breasts that pressed against restraint like silicone torpedoes. Joan felt the twinge. *How much of our humor is boob humor. How awkward it will be.*

"Where do you suppose she buys bras," Joan said.

"They probably make them out of the material you broads don't use," John said.

"Maybe they're falsies," Joan said.

The steak came and they ate. Joan was funny and animated that night. The part of her that sat in the balcony and looked down was very impressed. *That's a hell of a performance she's putting on.* Joan drew strength out of the good performance.

For Ace the doubleness was more complicated. He was enjoying himself. He loved to see her talk and hear her laugh. He enjoyed being in the room when she talked on the phone, so he could hear the bubbling talk and see the brightness in her face when she laughed. And here she was antimated and lively and he felt the muscle-tightening physical sensation he had felt so often near her in the last twenty-five years. *Jesus Christ, can she be dying? Beautiful and funny and dying? And me laughing and making fun of people and eating my steak and drinking the beer, they always get it cold enough here, and not many places do, and at the same time I'm thinking about the cold beer I'm thinking about her having cancer and dying. It can't be true and yet it can be and may be and I can't do anything about it. Thinking about it is not a plus. Avoid that.* And so his life went along on two parallel levels. He enjoyed the steak, he liked the laughter. He kidded with his friends. He watched the sports events. And he feared the death of his wife. And he did these things simultaneously. Amazing.

Sunday, April 20

Joan woke up at four-thirty. It was still dark. *Today I go. I've got all those tapes to do.* She got up and went to the kitchen. She made some instant coffee, took out a bran muffin, and sat down at the table in the family room and began to tape. Ace had set it up for her the night before: Daniel's little white Panasonic tape recorder with the built-in mike. Extra cassettes stacked beside it, a long yellow heavy-duty extension cord, three-pronged, the kind he used with his power tools, stretched across the table and plugged into the wall. It overpowered the little recorder. She almost smiled. *He couldn't use a regular extension, a little white one.*

There was something about the taping. About knowing that her voice would be heard in days ahead by people who didn't know. That when the tapes played things would have happened to her. In her robe and with her hair up and her face smeared with cream, she sat in the darkened family room and began to talk to the students who wouldn't hear her until Monday at the earliest.

"Hello, ladies. I'm not going to be able to be with you for a few days. I'm having some surgery and it can't be avoided. Big Bobbo will be bringing these tapes in . . ." and she went on. Child Growth and Development, and Reading Methods, one week's worth of each, six hours of tape. As she talked her voice got hoarse, there were pauses, long sighs, stretches when the voice quavered. The sky lightened. The sun came up. The dog moseyed out of the bedroom and sat at her foot and panted at her. Ace woke up and made coffee in the kitchen. The boys appeared, Ace made them breakfast. Still she taped. "Now," she said at the still, white recorder, "we can look at the Orton Method."

In the kitchen he was angry. *None of the other turkeys down there would do this. Who gives a shit about the Orton Method? Spend her last day busting her ass for Ding Dong School. They wouldn't do it for her.* A professor at a large urban university, he was continuously amazed at the amount of intrusive busy-work Joan encountered.

"You do this for those assholes," he said.

She stopped the tape. "Please don't," she said. "I do this for me and the kids. I love those students. They need this course. They have a month, most of them, till graduation and they will be all screwed up if they don't get this. I need to do this."

"I know. I know." He shook his head and went away. It was beyond him. His concerns were more primitive. They didn't extend much beyond the campfire. *That's their problem. Let the goddamned school thrash that out. They'll graduate them.*

He half knew that his anger went beyond that. He hated the intrusion of alien factors in the family. All his life he'd left his work at the office. Even now he never wrote on weekends or in the evening. He resented the fact that she allowed the job in. He knew also that the taping was something she should do for herself. Like everything else she did, it was a way of managing a slippery universe. Imposing some order on a situation that threatened dissolution. And he knew if she weren't doing this they'd have to find something else to fill the day. Sitting together, watching the clock tick toward check-in time, would be crippling.

So he went away and said no more and regretted saying anything, but his fury toward the school, a fury deflected from her by his affection and by her need, simmered without outlet. He relished the fantasy that when he brought the tapes in someone would give him trouble. *When this is over maybe I'll go down and kick in their fucking library.*

In the late morning Norma called to say that Gretchen Benjamin was away, at the Cape, and wouldn't be back. There was no way they could talk. Joan was disappointed, but somehow a numbness had set in and the latest disappointment seemed somehow inevitable and right. She never did get a chance until after it was over to talk with a woman who'd had breast surgery. The comfort that would have provided was not to be. In early afternoon the traffic in the kitchen and family room was interfering with her lectures, so she took the recorder into the bedroom, where she could finish it up. He watched the Seattle Supersonics and the Chicago Bulls on television.

Brent Musburger's voice, as he called the play by play, was full of confidence and pleasure. Certain and permanent, as if growing old and getting sick didn't happen. And Slick Watts, moving with the ball, his headband garish on his shaven head, framed in the television tube, resurrected by instant replay, seemed immortal. It was an illusion and he knew it, but it was illusion to which he gave himself fully. Appreciating Tom Boerwinkle's pick-and-roll with Jerry Sloan, caring about the execution of a game. *The results of games are mostly produced by the players. Maybe that's part of the charm.*

At half time he went and looked in at her and she was crying. It scared him. He didn't know what to say. What could he do to change the way it was? What solace could he bring? The fear overwhelmed the sorrow. He didn't feel sorry for her at that moment, he felt frightened that he'd fail. *Jesus I wish it was time for the hospital.*

He sat on the edge of the bed and put his hand on her back between her shoulder blades and moved it in a slow circle. He didn't say anything. It was the first time he'd seen her cry.

"I can't stand it," she said. Her voice was thick and teary. "I can't stand it."

"We have to," he said. "We haven't got any other option." He was uncomfortably conscious of how trite it was, what he'd said. How like the dialogue in an unsuccessful movie. He had always said we, from the beginning. Both on impulse and by design, he had included himself in the sickness; he hoped it made her less alone.

"I don't want them to chop me up a piece at a time. A boob, then the other boob, the ovaries, what else. I don't want to live like that. I would rather die."

"We don't look down that road. There's nothing there," he said. "We just take it as it comes. And we don't guess and we don't think about the next thing. We just look right at this thing. Today. Now. We don't think about maybe, and what if."

"You won't let them chop me up, Ace." Her face was red and distorted with crying and she pressed it into the mattress muffling what she said. His hand moved around steadily between her shoulder blades.

"No," he said. "I won't let them. I promise. If I have to I will kill you."

"Promise."

"I promise. You know I will. You know I can do what I have to do." *I can too.* He had thought of that already and knew that it was serious and knew that she meant it and knew that he did, but he also knew in the other ironic part of him that was open-shuttered and recording that this was melodrama of an intense kind. *I could never put this dialogue down in fiction,* he thought. *It is very hokey.*

"But that's tomorrow, or next month, and we don't think about that. We've got to concentrate on what we know. Today you check in. Tomorrow you have tests, Tuesday you have tests, and Wednesday you have surgery and maybe a mastectomy. That's what we know and that's all we know and we gotta concentrate on that and not speculate. We have to, otherwise we go crazy."

"I know."

As he talked his hand moved in the same steady circle between her shoulder blades. She had stopped crying.

"I think you ought to get ready to go," he said.

And now she wanted to. But there were things she had yet to do. "Pretty soon," she said.

He left her alone and went back to the porch to watch the second half. It had been harrowing, but he'd done it. He hadn't failed. What he'd said was what he should have said. *It was hardly fresh material,* he thought. *But it was true.* Throughout that spring he noticed how commonplace were the things of suffering and fear, and how commonplace their defense. *Remarkable.*

In the middle of the third quarter, with the score 69 to 63,

Seattle, Sharon and Mike appeared at the front door with a box of candy. As he opened the door he said to himself, *Not this time,* and stood in the open doorway and smiled but didn't invite them in.

"Joan's asleep right now," he said. "She's going to the hospital for a little surgery later today and needs to rest."

They gave him the box of candy. Mike asked for and got a glass of milk. They thanked him for Joan's help, and it was clear they wanted to stay.

"Okay, kids," Ace said. "Thanks for the candy. We'll see you." He gently herded them toward the door as he spoke. When they were gone he ate two pieces of candy and went back to watch the rest of the game.

Chapter 13 ~

Joan cleaned up the loose ends. She called her aunt in western Mass. Joan was fond of Virginia. She didn't tell her what was happening. She just called to talk, to hear Virginia's voice. Joan's parents were dead; Virginia was almost all that was left of family outside of Ace and the boys. Joan was never sure what prompted the call, a sense perhaps of I'm-never-coming-home-from-this, a desire to talk with Virginia before she went. *I want to talk with her before I go,* was all she could articulate. *But what does go mean?* she thought. *Does it mean before I go to the hospital or before I cash in the old chips? I don't know. But I want to talk.*

She called several people that afternoon, old friends she hadn't talked with lately, and talked and said goodbye without telling them. And then it was time. *Okay,* she said to herself, *okay I've put my house in order. I want to go. The house is clean, the tapes are done. The phone calls are made. Now I want to go.*

Monday was David's sixteenth birthday. She wouldn't be there. Holidays meant a lot to her, birthdays and Christmas particularly. They were important. She wrote a small birthday card with a poem, a variation on the roses-are-red-violets-are-blue theme, as she always did. She wrote one for her father-in-law, whose birthday was also April 21, and what she called unbirthday cards for Ace and Daniel. She gave all of them but Ace's to Ace to give out the next day. His she slipped under the spread onto his pillow, so he'd find it when he went to bed.

As she wrote the cards here eyes filled. *Jesus, is this it? Write the old cards and you won't be here for the kid's birthday. Why is this happening to me? How can I take it? How can I endure what's happening to me, what's ahead of me? How can I let them do this horrendous thing to my bod? Why can't I stop it?* And she could hear his voice. *'We'll deal with what we have to, we won't look down the road, we won't waste time asking why. We'll do what we have to.'* And she pushed back the self-pity. She talked to herself. *This is the right thing to do. This has happened to you and you must take it. You must hang on like hell. You must hope the surgery does the trick and the cancer hasn't spread. You mustn't get bogged down in why me. You must not.* But *Jesus, where the hell had that thing come from?* And she knew what he'd say to that, even though she'd never asked him. He'd say, *'It doesn't matter where it came from. It only matters that it's here and we have to get rid of it.'* And now she wanted very much to go. *I want to get the hell out of this house and get this the hell over with.*

They had agreed that it would be better if the boys didn't go with them to the hospital. She said goodbye to them at home. At twelve, Daniel was very loving and huggy. He gave her a large hand-drawn card to take with her to the hospital. It had many "loves" written on it. Joan thanked him profusely, thinking as she did, *Jesus maybe I'm going overboard because Dave hasn't given me a card and he'll feel bad.* It was harder for David to be demonstrative at sixteen. At any age he had always been a very interior person. They parted without tears, but with little laughter either and with faces that revealed that what they were doing was hard.

Driving to the hospital with her suitcases in the back of the station wagon, he thought of the times he'd driven her before. Twice, for the babies, *beginnings and endings,* he thought. He did not share the thought with her. *When bathos can be avoided it should be.* Union Hospital was no more than a mile from home and the drive was brief. In the parking lot they met June Crumrine, who did volunteer work at the hospital. They stopped and talked. Ace had Joan's luggage in hand. Joan was obviously checking into the hospital. June could obviously see that. June obviously wondered why, but was obviously not going to ask. Joan obviously was not going to say. It was one of the clumsier moments of the period.

As they sat in the admitting office and waited while the forms were typed, he said, "You gotta start telling people. Poor June didn't know what the hell was happening. She's a good friend and she's confused."

"Would it have been easier on her if I'd said I have breast cancer and I'm going in for a mastectomy?"

"No, I suppose it wouldn't. But you can't keep this quiet. It hasn't even happened yet and half of Lynnfield knows you're in the hospital or having surgery or have a lump. You can't keep it quiet. You have too many friends. You know too many people. I could come in and have my head removed and keep it a secret. But you — it's going to be known."

"Well, let's be sure. Let's keep it quiet until we're sure."

"How about the special people? Ganems, for instance. Can I tell them?"

"Yes, but wait till we know. Unless it comes up for some reason. You know the people that I love. You tell them when you think you should."

Being in the hospital was for both of them a relief. They had plugged into the process and the process would carry them for a while. It was as if they'd finished a long journey. A candy striper led them to Joan's room. Eliopoulos had gotten her the private room, West Wing, second floor at the end of the corridor over-looking a small side street where the homes had gardens behind them. There was a private bath and a television. And a phone. Ace showed her how the TV worked. She unpacked. In her suit-case, slipped into a side pocket, was a card from David which showed a small boy hugging a puppy. "Without you I'm noth-ing," the card said. "I miss you already." Joan's eyes filled and she showed it to Ace. *God,* she thought, *that is a grabber.* He read it without comment and felt his throat tighten.

"I'll call you," she said, her voice a little thick, "when I know the visiting hours."

"It doesn't matter," he said. "They haven't got enough bodies to keep me out when I want to come in. Visiting hours or not."

He gave her a batch of magazines he'd bought her. And then there was nothing to do. He wanted to get out of there. He wanted to run. She felt herself coil and tighten in. She wanted him to go. They were ill at ease. In twenty years he had never been ill at ease with her. In twenty years he'd never wanted to run away from her. They hugged each other.

"Some nice sabbatical I'm having," he said.

"Too bad this didn't happen last year," she said. "You could have skipped a bunch of classes."

"David has to get the bus at seven-thirty," she said. "And Dan at quarter of eight. Dan always has his breakfast while he's watching 'Beaver.'"

"Yeah," he said. "I know all about that."

"And you take my tapes tomorrow to Endicott. Class starts at nine."

"I know that."

"And you know where to go."

"Yeah."

"Okay."

They stepped away from each other. He went to the door. "I love you," he said.

"Love," she said.

"If an intern makes a move on you, tell him your husband's going to kill him."

"Maybe I will and maybe I won't," she said.

He went out the door and left the hospital.

Joan closed the door and looked out the window. The room was bright and pleasant. The hospital was very quiet. Sunday afternoon quiet. She sat in the chair and read a little bit in the magazines that he'd brought her, but it was hard to concentrate. She looked at her watch. Actually it was David's watch and much too big for her wrist, but she couldn't stand not knowing the time and she'd borrowed it for the occasion. Four-thirty. *A little early to put on the jammies and hop into bed.* She got up and looked at her face in the mirror. She redid her eye makeup. She looked at her breasts; *even. One on each side.* She sat in the chair by the window and read *People* magazine and listened to the sounds of trays clattering and nurse's aides talking and supper being served. She was hungry. Every once in a while she opened her door and looked out. No one paid her any attention, so she closed it again and read on. *You know how nurses are. They don't like it if you're naggy or demanding. You've got to be Harriet Humble while you're in here, kiddo, you gotta be real nice to everybody.*

Chapter 14 ⌒

HE DROVE HOME balanced between relief and desolation. His responsibilities for her were shared now. She was in the hands of professionals. *There's more to it than that, though,* he thought. *It's the paternalism, too. A duly constituted authority has appeared on the scene. The beds are made square and the floors are clean and supper comes in balanced variety, planned by a dietician, properly nourishing, with the calories all counted. A clean well-lighted place.* He felt no guilt over his relief. He knew he needed it. He knew his reactions were human, all of them. Objectively he was fascinated to watch what happened to him in extremity. *If there's such a thing as the essential self,* he thought, as he pulled out onto Lynnfield Street, *I am now in touch with it. This is real.*

It was the implacable reality of it all that startled him regularly. She couldn't die and yet she might. He could not lose her and yet he might. *Death isn't the mother of beauty. It's just death. The realist bastard there is.* It was a reality he faced with a desolation too profound to speak, even to himself. And he felt himself press against it with a soundless inarticulate certainty that he

could stand the desolation. *I have two sons.* He said to himself.
I have two sons.

He pulled into his driveway under the thirty-year-old sugar
maple that was starting to green. In March they had tapped it,
and taken out enough sap for three quarts of maple syrup. He'd
closed the hole with a plug made from a maple branch and already the tree was beginning to heal around it.

Inside the boys seemed easy and unsuspicious. Both had been
in the hospital at one time or another and it held no mysteries for
them. But he didn't want to be home. It was too bright, too
pleasant, and he knew the bright pleasantness might be illusory.
He was hard pressed to be easy and unconcerned.

"I gotta go tell Jude that Mom's all settled in, and where she
is and stuff," he said.

Dave nodded. Dan said, "Okay."

He walked across the street and into Judy's house. Her kids
were in the den watching TV. Judy was in the kitchen.

"John's got hockey," she said. "How is she?"

"Good," he said. "She's in West Wing Two. Private room,
which is good."

"Is she okay?"

"Yeah. She's scared. She's scared most that they'll keep cutting away at her."

Judy started to cry. She said, "Oh, Ace."

"I won't let them cut away a piece at a time. I promised her
that." He felt the old feeling. The achiness in the throat, the
voice becoming hoarse, and he started to cry too. It was the only
time.

"Jesus Christ, Ace, I'm supposed to be consoling you."

He turned from her, embarrassed that he'd cried and that his
nose was runny.

"You're doing swell, Jude," he said. He got a paper towel from
her towel rack and blew his nose.

From the front door a voice said, "Hello" and Bill Ganem came in with two of his children.

Judy, red-eyed and weeping, said, "Hi, Bill." Ace blew his nose again.

"Is Eileen with you?" Ace said.

"She's in New Jersey with Barbara and Billy. I was up at my mother's and thought I'd stop off on my way home."

He knew something was wrong. "Where's John and J?" he said. Bill had known them since they were all eighteen, and he'd always called Joan by her first initial, no one could remember why now, if there had even been a reason.

"John's got hockey," Judy said. She looked at Ace. "Why don't Cindy and Sally go watch TV with my kids," Jude said.

Bill shooed his daughters into the den. When they were gone Ace said, "This is going to be tough to hear and you don't have to have any reactions to it. I wouldn't know what to say if I were you and it's okay. Joan's in the hospital, she found a lump in her left breast and it's probably cancerous and they will probably have to take the breast."

Bill's round Arabic face darkened and the lines deepened and pain showed. It was one of his charms, a capacity for empathy that one rarely encounteed. *Sometimes people are only startled,* Ace thought, *but he hurts too. Like Jude.*

"Jesus Christ," Bill said. "Are they sure?"

"No. But they're pretty sure. They'll do some tests Monday and Tuesday, and biopsy her Wednesday. If it's malignant they'll take the breast before she wakes up."

"Jesus Christ. I won't tell Eileen until Wednesday. Will you call me and tell me as soon as you know?"

"Yes."

"If I tell Eileen she'll be upset as a bastard. I won't tell her until you're sure. She'll want to come right home."

"Tell her not to. There's no need."

"She'll be punchy coming out of anesthesia," Judy said. "She'll have a lot of medication and she won't feel like visitors for at least a day, maybe more."

Ace got two beers out of Judy's refrigerator and gave one to Bill. They drank the beers and talked a little and the pain never left Bill's face. When the beer was gone he took the kids and left.

"I bet he's glad he stopped off," Ace said.

"Poor Bill."

"When Joan has the surgery I'd like you to special her."

"Of course."

"I think she needs a woman, and I want to be sure someone's there."

"Yes, that will be good. That way if she is in pain I can go right down and get the medication and make sure she gets it as soon as she can have it."

"She worrying about looking bad in your eyes when she's coming to and acting crazy."

"That's ridiculous."

"I know. But she worries about stuff like that."

They were quiet.

"Can I count on you to special her as long as she needs it," he said. "I don't mean like four hours, I mean as long as it takes?"

"Oh, Ace, of course."

"I expect to pay."

"Oh, Ace, fuck off."

"No, I mean that. There's no reason to not get paid."

"Shut up."

"Jude, you're supposed to be cheering me up and making me feel better."

"Then don't be an asshole."

"We'll talk about it later. How did John react?"

"He couldn't believe it. He kept saying 'Joan?' I mean it was like, Joan's too lively and, you know, healthy."

"Vital," Ace said.

"Yes, that's it."

"Words are my game," Ace said.

"He couldn't get over not knowing last night. I think he felt bad about that, but he understood why."

It was starting to get dark outside Joan's window and she couldn't see the neat yards in back of the small houses very well anymore. A nurse opened the door and stuck her head in. She was a young nurse with long brown hair and sharp pretty features. She scanned the room and saw no tray.

"Have you had supper?"

Joan shook her head. "No, I haven't," she said, trying to keep any hint of martyrdom out of her voice.

"Well, that's a mistake; somebody hasn't been on the job. I'll get supper right up to you. Why don't you pull that table over and I'll be right back with a tray."

Her head disappeared and Joan heard her rubber-soled shoes thumping down the corridor. She pulled the table over and swung it around in front of her. The nurse came back in with the supper tray, the white skirt of her uniform whipping as she walked.

Supper was a slice of roast veal, whipped potatoes, carrots, and cottage cheese with pineapple. Joan ate it all. *My stomach doesn't know I have cancer. I'm eating like a cow. I'm also having continual diarrhea from fear and losing weight anyway. I may as well eat while I can.*

After she had been discovered nurses dropped in all evening.

This is a terrific group of nurses, Joan thought. *But it's my ailment too. There's something about breast cancer and mastectomy that brings women closer to me. There's a feeling almost of sisterhood. My God, me and Ti-Grace Atkinson — Sisterhood.* But it was there, a sense of specialness, of a woman's mystery, that men, even Ace, could not entirely share. Mingled with the fear and the terrors of disfigurement and dissolution, there was a sense of new doors opening, and a new sense of femalehood. *If I make this, I'll have to think about that.* For now she knew that her care was warm and supportive and superlative. She discovered that she didn't know how nurses were at all.

Sunday night Ace called his mother and father and told them what he knew. They were calm about it. His mother knew several people who'd had mastectomies years ago and were fine. He felt somehow calmer talking to them. *Some things you never lose,* he thought afterward, remembering his mother's calm voice on the phone. *Parents still make you feel secure. We never completely give up on Santa Claus.*

Chapter 15 ⌒

MONDAY, APRIL 21 and Tuesday were a blur of tests. Body and bone scans were simply x-rays of various kinds from various angles. They were painless. Monday afternoon Edgar Mitchell, a plastic surgeon, dropped by and sat in the yellow plastic-covered armchair by the window and talked with Joan about reconstructive surgery.

"John asked me to stop by and talk with you," he said.

It took Joan a moment to realize that John was Dr. Eliopoulos.

"Oh yes, I remember asking him about reconstruction."

"Well, it is entirely possible," Mitchell said. "I have not done it yet myself, but I would very much like to. It's a very interesting trick."

"They implant something, is that right?"

"Yes, a small sack of inert jell is anchored and the new skin is grafted over it. The jell can't drift, not like an injection. It is, as far as I've heard, entirely safe, and not a very big operation."

"How about the nipple?"

"That can be done too; not everyone bothers, but if you wanted it, we could graft skin from, say, the labia and rebuild the nipple and its areola."

"When you say it's not a big operation, how big?"

"Perhaps overnight."

"How soon could it be done?"

"Oh, a year or so after the original incision has healed and everything is in order."

"I don't have to decide now?"

"No. I will talk to John about this and when he does the surgery he will keep it in mind. If he has to take the breast he will have reconstruction in mind."

Mitchell was a stocky, solid, Scotch-looking man with dark hair speckled gray and dark-rimmed glasses. He smoked a pipe.

During the two test days Fred Shmaese dropped in as well. Shmaese was an oncologist from Lynnfield. They knew each other slightly at the time, and he came, informally, to talk with Joan. He sat on the edge of the bed, a solemn, formal, skillful man with strong opinions, and talked with her about breast cancer, and mastectomy and tumors in general and also about the state of education and the direction the world found itself running in.

Like Dr. Mitchell, Shmaese did not say she was going to undergo mastectomy, but it was tacitly assumed, and the calmness of the discussion with Fred, as it had been with Mitchell, was to make the illness and the surgical act seem more ordinary. The focus of all conversations on what-we-do-after-the-breast-is-gone. When the time came she was ready and fully prepared to wake up from anesthesia with the breast gone. Whether that was an artfully orchestrated preparation for surgery or not she was never sure. But by Tuesday night she was looking long past the surgery on Wednesday to concern for lymph node involvement. Her concern was steadily less with her breast and more with her life.

Monday morning Ace took the tapes and drove to Endicott

College. Joan's class was in a small white clapboard building surrounded by trees on the east slope of a hill. It seemed isolated from the rest of the campus. There were three classrooms in the building, one devoted to a children's school and two for college courses. He went in carrying her two briefcases and the tape recorder. The department supervisor was a woman, the students were women. It was a very female place and he was struck by that. He was a bit out of place there. Judy Martin was uneasy with him, attempting to banter with him in a light girlish way. *Is it because I'm male?* he thought, *or does she always do June Allyson? I hope not. She doesn't have the build for it.* In the classroom the girls looked puzzled. And he felt a little outsized, inappropriate.

"As you may have noticed," he said. "I am not Joan Parker."

No one smiled. They all stared at him solemnly.

"Mrs. Parker had to have some surgery," he went on, "and she has asked me to cover for her for a bit. She's taped her lectures and I'm here to play them and assist in whatever way I can. Which is not much, because I know less than you do about the subject."

A hand went up. "What about the final exam?"

"We'll worry about that when it's time to. You won't suffer for it, whatever the situation."

Another hand. "When will she be back?"

"How quickly you tire of me," he said. "I don't know. We'll have to wait and see."

"Could you tell us where she is, so we can send her a card?"

"Sure." He wrote the address on the board.

"Can we visit?"

"Not yet. I'll tell you when. Any other questions?"

There were none. "Now the good news. There will be no class Wednesday." He took an extension cord from one of the briefcases and plugged in the tape recorder. "Okay," he said. "Here we go."

Joan's voice came from the recorder. "Good morning, ladies . . ." He realized he could not stand to listen. "I'll be back in a while," he said over the tape, and headed for the door. Her voice had a hoarse faintly shaky sound to it, as it drifted out with him. He shut the door behind him.

As Joan waited outside of X-ray she thought about James Stacey. Sitting alone her first day in the hospital and reading *People* magazine she had come across a picture of James Stacey, young movie star, who had been badly maimed in an accident, losing a leg and an arm. The picture stayed with her. There he was on one leg with one arm balancing on skis on a steep slope. The empty leg of his ski pants was pinned up and the poles were of an unusual kind that would help him balance, and on his face was a broad smile. *Just the biggest smilingest face,* she thought, *out on the goddamned slopes in Vermont or someplace and he's obviously having a hell of a good time.* She remembered her talk with Ace about not being hacked to bits, and his promise. *Well, maybe I could take some hacking. Look at Stacey. He took a hell of a lot and was still extracting pleasure from life. Maybe if they do have to cut away at me. Maybe if it's spread out I could go on. I could have some fun. I would have a different kind of life. I would have to set an example for people. I'll have to be a different kind of Joan. A Joan people don't like to look at. A Joan people would feel funny about. People would be saying, 'Jesus-I-don't-want-that-to-happen-to-me.' But maybe I can use myself as an example. Maybe I can find a way to have some kind of dignity and a way of life that is somehow productive even though it may be in a whole other direction than I ever intended to go. Maybe I can do that. Could do that if it happened.* It always struck her that she owed James Stacey something and they'd never met and he'd never know.

For such introspection there was little time, however. Every nurse who came in to escort her to X-ray or take a blood sample or take her temperature or bring her lunch went far beyond the necessities of her work. They talked with Joan. They initiated conversation. They told her about aunts and mothers and sisters and former patients who had undergone breast surgery and whose recovery had been comfortable and complete. *It's like everyone loves me. I feel, for God's sake, I feel loved in here.*

And Benny, the respiration therapist. He was there from the first day. Under the stress of panic in Dr. Eliopoulos' office that first day, she had smoked two cigarettes which Ace had bummed for her from the receptionist. Under the impression that she was a heavy smoker, Eliopoulos had prescribed presurgical respiration therapy. Benny was a short heavy cheerful man who wheeled his respiration machine in three times a day on Monday and another three on Tuesday and talked and joked with her, and taught her how to use the machine, and seemed to care how she felt, not professionally but in fact. They talked a bit of her fears, although mostly she breathed in and out according to his instructions and he talked to her. He talked of certain postsurgical black periods in his own life and how he'd gotten through them. He was a very kind man and Joan looked forward to his visits.

On the floor below was Gerry Wilkinson, a neighbor who had the previous week fallen from a stepladder and broken her ankle. It was a bad break for a woman in her fifties and she would be a long time bedridden. Joan went down to visit her frequently during her free moments and drew strength from Gerry's calm acceptance of what might be a crippling injury.

"I will pray for you, Joan," Gerry had said. "And I will ask Warren and the children to pray for you too." Gerry's God was Catholic and immediate, a God whose eye was on the fall of a sparrow and she gained strength from Him. Joan didn't believe, but she gained strength in some odd way from Gerry's belief. It was comforting to think that people were praying for her, to a God they believed in. Joan always felt calmer after talking with Gerry Wilkinson.

Across the hall Mrs. Bacheldor and her roommate Helga were good to talk with. Mrs. Bacheldor promised to put Joan in touch with a friend who had survived a mastectomy in flourishing health. She promised to put Joan in touch with her after the operation.

While Joan's tapes were running, Ace drove into Beverly, looking for a cup of coffee. He found a Dunkin' Donut stand and got a large black to go. He drove to a drugstore and bought a copy of the Boston *Globe*. He drove back to the campus and sat in the car and drank the coffee and read the paper. The children from the Lab School kindergarten came out while he sat there and played and ran about, under the supervision of a head teacher and some students. He noticed that several of the children stayed by themselves and he felt bad for them.

Joan's first class ended at ten-fifteen and he went in to shut off the tapes. The students were already starting to file out. He smiled at them vaguely as they passed, his mind busy with other things, impatient that he must be here.

During the second class he drove down along the shore road into Manchester and back, sightseeing, listening to the radio, remembering when they were very young and not yet married how the two of them had driven down to a club in Magnolia to hear Sarah Vaughan. He noticed that thinking about it neither increased nor decreased the ache of anxiety in him. Generally he didn't like to remember the time before they were married, for those were times when he didn't have her and she was still uncertain if she would marry him and he felt retrospective fear that a matter of such moment to him had been entrusted to such unskilled hands as his had been at nineteen. *I could have lost her.*

What would have happened to me if I had lost her? If I lose her now at least I'll have had her. I'll have had eighteen years and eight months. And now I have my sons. Then I would have had nothing and I wouldn't have even been what I am now. I had potential but I was an awful turkey. She took a chance and she knew it. She was always more pragmatic than I was. She calculated and weighed and said, 'Okay, it's my best shot.' And she did it, and she was right. But it was a gamble and at that time in her life she wasn't a gambler. Jesus Christ. It's like remembering when you were shot at and missed.

Thinking of the past depressed him. And he drove in silence, trying to concentrate simply on the music and the August houses that rolled by on the winding road. *Thinking of the future isn't an upper either. Carpe diem, babe.*

It was nearly lunchtime when Joan heard him coming down the hall. She knew from the time that he was stopping off directly on the way home from Endicott. When he came in the room he was dressed as he was always dressed. Blue corduroy Levi jacket, blue Adidas with a white stripe, sunglasses. He was carrying her briefcases.

"They prefer me," he said. "They claim I'm better looking and smarter and they want me to stay."

"How did it go?"

"Fine."

"Did they ask much about me?"

"Yeah, some. Where were you, could they send a card, what were visiting hours, like that."

"What did you tell them?"

"I told them you had to have some surgery, that you were here, and that I'd let them know about visiting hours and when they could come."

"You didn't tell them about the mastectomy?"

"No."

"Did anyone ask what the surgery was?"

"No."

"Did anyone tell you I was wonderful?"

"No."

"Oh."

He unpacked the briefcases and set the tape recorder up on the windowsill so that she could do more taping if she had a chance. A nurse came in with lunch under the covered dishes on a tray. *Served that way it always looks tasty,* he thought, *even when it isn't.* Joan asked about a low-calorie diet.

"I'm eating like a pig in here, Norah," she said. "I'll look like the Goodyear blimp."

"I'll ask the dietician to come by later," Norah said. "She can help you work out what you want. Remember you'll need a lot of nourishment after surgery. This isn't a time to starve yourself."

"I know," Joan said. "But I'm so hungry. I'm hungry all the damn time."

"Now you know how I feel," Ace said. "That's the story of my life. I've been hungry and thirsty and horny since I was eight months old."

"No wonder you wanted a private room," Norah said. All of them laughed. The nurse left. He reached over and took the cover off one of the dishes. Tuna salad. There were two pickles on the plate with the salad. He took one. "Why don't I run down and get a sandwich and a coffee from the cafeteria and bring it up and eat lunch with you?" he said.

"Okay, but make it quick; I'm having a hunger tantrum now."

He got his sandwich and a black coffee to go and carried it back up to her room. They ate in relative quiet. There was little to say. But they had been together long, and having nothing to say was not awkward. When they were through he left.

"I'll come back around suppertime with the kids and we'll, like, have supper with you."

"I don't think you're supposed to bring food in."

"No, we'll eat at home, but early, so we can come down and be with you while you eat. I assume you have stuff this afternoon."

"Yes."

"Okay, see ya."

"Bye-bye."

She heard his step recede down the corridor and heard him joke with Nurse Pike, the head nurse, as he passed the charge desk, and then he was gone. He always made her feel stronger. She knew he could do everything that had to be done. *Absolutely everything,* she thought. *Take my courses, take care of the kids, whatever. He is always there. Always.* There was about him a quality of massive stability. It was hard to remember when he hadn't been there.

A half hour after Ace left, Dr. Helen Walsh, the anesthesiologist, came to visit. She asked Joan about allergies and loose teeth and things anesthesiologists need to know. But she had also come to talk. For Joan she was a pleasure, a doctor, a woman, and a warm concerned person.

"This is Connie Coward, Helen. I'm afraid of pain."

"There will be medication," Helen said. "We can deal with pain all right."

"Will I be crazy, screaming, bothering people? I don't want to do badly."

Helen shook her head. "You won't be. It won't be that bad. Some discomfort yes, but not pain. Nothing medication won't get you through fine. You really needn't worry about that."

It was true what Jude had told her, and now Helen had said it and Joan believed it. *She seems to respect me. That helps. Her respect is helpful.*

In the late afternoon Judy and John came to visit. John was a hockey coach, a muscular jock-ethic man who used humor as they themselves did as a means of concealment and a tool of communication.

For Joan he was in a way the symbolic male, the one who had to accept her loss of sexuality on behalf of all males. She dreaded the first meeting, fearing what she might sense, afraid he might feel something he could not conceal, conscious that she must put him at once at ease, nervous that perhaps she couldn't. It was a real hurdle for her, and an indication of her postoperative state of mind. Her breast was still there, but already she acted as if it were gone.

As she waited for them to come she reflected partially about the degree to which being the object of sexual desire was one base of her relationship with men. It was not that she slept around or wanted to, though she'd always been as she said to Ace, "curious." She had been only with her husband and it seemed very likely now that she only would be. But being desired seemed, now that she feared she wouldn't be, to have been a larger part in her male friendships than she had thought. It was not so much that she perceived desire from them as that she felt herself desirable. John, because he was in some ways an extreme of masculinity, loomed to her as a test case. If John were not visibly put off, perhaps men wouldn't be. Ace, for all his maleness, was no test. They both knew that. His feelings were irrevocable, as fixed as the sun.

The thing she had been saying to people about her upcoming surgery was, "Easy come, easy go." And she used it on John and Jude when they came. It was a good start and John seemed to like the remark and treat her as before. He did not seem to see her as grotesque or as grotesque-to-be. If he did he concealed it so well that she got no sign of it. They talked as easily and humorously, their humor full of put-downs, as they always did. When they left her she was buoyed by their visit. No one seemed

horrified, no one was full of pity. Everyone expected her to recover and be what she had been.

Monday afternoon David went to the library and looked up
breast cancer. He'd had the feeling when his mother and father
went yesterday to the hospital that more than a simple cyst was
involved.

*Dad didn't seem like a man driving his wife to the hospital
for a little cyst operation. He seemed like a man driving his wife
to the hospital with breast cancer.*

He spent an hour in the town library researching breast cancer
and when he left he was certain his mother had it. But he said
nothing to anyone.

In Tuesday's mail there had come, also, a note from Billy
Ganem — she had known him since she had known Ace — and
the letter, like John and Jude's visit, helped her through another day. It was an honest expression of pain at her illness and
of love that would endure beyond any illness. It surely had been
a hard letter to write. Billy, like John and like Ace, for that
matter, was a product of the fifties, and of assumption about male
behavior that limited displays of emotion. It was another piece
in the structure of support that built up around her that spring,
a structure as important to her as the medical skills that the
hospital supplied and the capacities of Eliopoulos's hands.

The boys and Ace came and stayed with her at supper, and
watched television for some time afterward. It was little different
than it would have been at home except that they all had to
watch the same program, and Ace, who hated almost all television equally, got restless and walked around the room and up
and down the corridors and bitched about the programming. At
home he could retire to another room. Dan called weather and
time on Joan's phone, fascinated with a private phone of one's
own.

Tuesday night they brought her an assortment of movie fan

magazines. She had a passion for fan magazines but was embarrassed to buy them. She read them only at the beauty parlor.

"The clerk looked at me kind of funny," Ace said when he gave her the magazines. "I bought one of every kind they had, except a whole issue devoted to Bobby Sherman."

Dave said, "You don't look like a teeny-bopper."

Dan said, "How about a Big Bopper," and everyone laughed.

Ace said, "There used to be a rock-and-roll singer named the Big Bopper."

"How about Whale Bopper?" Dan said.

"Want to hear my Big Bopper impression?" Ace said.

"No."

The kids fought a bit over what program to watch, and at nine the security guard came around, carrying his time clock and nightstick, and said that visiting hours were over.

"Be sure to meet my class tomorrow," she said as they left.

"Of course," he said.

When she was alone at night Joan thought about Jerry Wilkinson and her prayers. *It must be a great comfort to have that kind of belief. I'm not sure I have no belief, but . . . I certainly don't have any belief in a benevolent God that's taking care of me, working out my life to the best advantage. What's that line that Ace uses? . . . The ways of the Lord are often dark but never pleasant. Who said that originally? I'll ask Ace. I know it's not his. Anyway I could make some kind of bargain. But with whom? Maybe if I became a believer again? If I believe and promise to believe always you'll make this just be breast cancer and spare the rest of my body. You can take the boob and give me the rest of my body. Balls. What kind of God is that who would say, "Oh, okay. We were going to infuse your entire body with cancer, but as long as you agree to believe in me, we won't. We'll just take one boob. I can't accept that God. If he's up there I decline to accept him anyway. That's no deal.*

She was watching the "Johnny Carson Show." The sound came from the small speaker by her bed, and it had fallen away and hung from its strap, turned away from her. She couldn't hear what was being said, just a low entertainment noise and Carson's face like a good-natured boyish Satan. *He seems so good a man. How could all those divorces have happened? Why can't he live with a wife? He can't quit smoking either. But I can. I have. And I can make that deal with myself. I've been backsliding, a cigarette here, a puff on someone's there. I'm not becoming a smoker again, but this situation makes smoking more needful. If I get out of this I won't be a smoker again ever. I won't start smoking a few cigarettes at parties and worrying about whether I'm creating lung cancer, and waking up with the terrible smoking taste in my mouth and be scared about that. I won't smoke again if I get out of this. That's a deal with me, not with God.*

The pact with herself was something that made sense to her, and yet she knew there was superstition involved as well. Though she never felt a benevolent God by her side she was never able entirely to rid herself of the feeling that something was out there. Some presence. *Maybe just a hangover from childhood belief,* she thought, *maybe superstition.* But there was a sense of someone out there to whom she addressed remarks now and then without thinking about it. "Listen, you've got to help me through this. I need help with this. Get me through tonight. Give me the strength to endure this." *Who am I talking to? Is it really God I'm talking to? I don't know.* She thought about mysticism. About contacting those who had died before her. Her mother, her father. She had some acquaintances who were very much convinced of the reality of such extracorporeal matters. *What do I do, start calling? Hello, out there. Hey, here I am. This is the time. This is when I need you.* It seemed laughable to her. She had to reject that. But she was looking for something and she very much wanted belief. She needed some pattern to this. Some way to order the experience and impose meaning on it. But she couldn't, and she had come, by late that night before surgery, to the simple realization that there was no order or meaning to it. She came to think of it as she did always thereafter as simply something that happened to her.

The meaning she found was in the mature and caring response of her children, the permanence of her husband, the commitment of her friends, the warm support of the nurses. *I don't know if there are any atheists in foxholes,* she thought as she drifted into sleep. *But there aren't any misanthropes, I'll bet.* Sleep was sound and dreamless. She had expected to spend the night awake and frightened. She did not. She couldn't remember getting a sleeping pill. She never did remember and she never thought to ask. *Maybe Valium,* she thought. *Maybe it's Valium that's putting me to sleep.*

Chapter 16 ~⌒

THEY WOKE HER very early for surgery. She was calm. Resigned. Not a lamb to slaughter. Simply one ready for what was to come. She was not frightened. *Valium, do your stuff,* she thought. But her calmness was more than just resignation. It was a kind of eagerness too. As she had wanted to come to the hospital Sunday, so now she wanted to get on with the surgery. *I have to come out of the other end of the tunnel. I have to get on with my life after this day and this surgery.* She wanted to begin that life. She wanted to get to a point of certainty. To know if she'd live.

She got up and did her face. Lipstick, blusher, eye makeup, mascara, eye liner. Her nails were done. She brushed her hair. She was very careful with her hair. Dr. Eliopoulos was quite a nice-looking man.

Norah came in and gave her a shot. "Just some medication to make you drowsy. Won't put you to sleep. Just make it easier for us to get you asleep in the OR."

Things did get a little drowsy then. Two nurses, Norah and Eunie, came in and shaved her chest.

"I don't want to spoil this," Joan said. "But I don't have any hair on my chest."

"We do it routinely," Norah said. "It's silly, but we always do it."

They put long white surgical stockings on her. *Like my mother used to wear,* she thought. *But they only came to your knees. Nice. Just like knee socks. Maybe I can keep these and wear them later. No, maybe not. Probably don't look good playing tennis in surgical stockings.*

One of the nurses said something about nail polish.

"What?"

"You'll have to remove your nail polish," the nurse said. Joan wasn't quite clear which nurse it was.

"Why," Joan said. "Why is that?"

"Oh, just take it off." The nurse handed her some polish remover.

"But I like it on there. I think it looks kind of neat."

"Well, the thing is they want to be able to tell if your nails turn blue. They have to be able to see that."

"Christ, I wish I hadn't asked," Joan said.

"And the makeup," someone said. A tissue appeared. "Okay, wipe it off."

Joan removed the makeup. The nurse washed her face.

Then she was moving. The bed was wheeled into the corridor. Benny was there, "You're going to be okay, okay." And into the elevator and down. Very down and then out into what seemed like a basement. Cinder-block walls painted bright green. A long corridor, other beds along the wall now and then. Nurses in green uniforms with skullcaps, and a strong sense of being deep underground. Windowless and silent. A different world right here on Lynnfield Street, next to the Shop Kwik Market that was always open. Even Christmas Day. And quite busy down there. The bed was parked next to the wall and Grace was there, a neighbor, but only a casual acquaintance. "Hi, Grace," and Grace startled. *It's my hat. I've got on one of the goddamned hats, and poor Grace doesn't know who the hell I am. Do I have on a hat?* "Grace, it is I, Joan Hall Parker."

And Grace, an operating-room assistant who cleans up, standing with her broom and saying, "Joan, what are you doing here?"

Good one, Grace. "I'm having some surgery, Grace. How've you been?"

Talk like they would have if they met over the potato bin at Star Market. "Good Joan, I've been good."

Then Helen Walsh was there, looking different with her hat and her stethoscope. She stayed. Joan was interested now. Asking questions. What was the IV for?

"In case we need to plug blood in right off, we can. We can keep a steady solution dripping in there. We can have access to your bloodstream instantly that way. Very handy."

"It is very bizarre," Joan said, "being down here. Very odd to think of the traffic going by right outside and people going to work and the children walking past to school, and down below here, with the white lights and the green walls."

"Oh, now, it's not that bad," Helen said.

"No, I don't mean it's bad. It's just so basementy otherworldly."

"I suppose it is," Helen Walsh said. "I get used to it. To me it's very routine. When we go into the OR I'll give you medication through the IV. You'll go to sleep almost instantly. You'll wake up in the recovery room and it will seem to you, you just went to sleep. I'll be there with you through the operation and I'll be with you when you wake up. I'll be right there with you and whatever needs to be done I'll see to it."

"I'm all right," Joan said. "I'm ready for whatever. It's okay."

They passed the time. They talked about Joan's teaching, about the Le Boyer birth-without-violence method. In the operating room there were big medical lights. *What makes them look medical. The indirectness? But they do.* The room seemed vaguely not square to her. Eliopoulos was there in his surgery suit. Several nurses. Helen Walsh near her head.

"Start counting backward from one hundred," Helen said.

"One hundred," Joan said.

"Good night," Helen said.

"Ninety-eight, ninety-seven . . ."

Joan was strapped to the table. They draped her with sheets, leaving open only the area on the left side of her chest. One sheet was draped vertically from a bar above her chest and acted as a sterile partition. At her head, behind the partition, Helen Walsh watched Joan closely. When the sheets were in place she administered 2 cc of Pentothal intravenously. It was a test dose. The room was quiet. Eliopoulos and the scrub nurse stood back a little, away from the table, in green caps and gowns, masked and sterile.

Joan's response to the test dose of Pentothal was right, and Helen Walsh gave her 400 milligrams. Joan lay motionless on the table. Helen brushed her eyelashes to see if there was reflex. There was none. With the circulating nurse standing by, Helen gave her pure oxygen through a face mask, watching the attached bag billow and shrink, and monitored her blood pressure, EKG, and other vital signs. The tiny blip on the display screen showed Joan's heartbeat steady. The room was quiet and the small beep of the monitor was loud, against the rush of the exhaust fan. Helen remembered surgery in ORs without the fans, when everyone was getting giddy from the anesthesia by the end of the surgery.

"She's fine," Helen murmured to the circulating nurse. She added halothane to the oxygen. The heart remained steady, the bag inflated and decreased with Joan's regular breath. If it be-came shallow Helen would assist by squeezing the bag. The circulating nurse washed the area of surgery with PhisoHex. Joan's left arm was stretched out and placed on a padded board. Her right arm the same with the IV tube in place and the blood-pressure cuff attached. Helen nodded at Eliopoulos.

Sterilized instruments on a sterilized surgical table stood ready. Before Joan had been wheeled in, the scrub nurse had laid them out, following the procedures card indexed for breast biopsy. Now John Eliopoulos took a surgical knife and made a two-inch incision in the skin of Joan's left breast above the lump, following the grain of the skin. After he made the cut he put the knife aside. The skin was assumed to be nonsterile and therefore the skin knife was no longer sterile. He used a pair of clamps to hold the lump and, guided by the feel through the new knife, he carefully cut out the lump. It appeared no different from the surrounding tissue. Joan's vital signs remained normal. Every five minutes Helen Walsh charted blood pressure, pulse, EKG. She was careful to remain behind the sterile barrier.

Eliopoulos took the small piece of tissue on a piece of gauze to the door of the room. He dropped it into the pathologist's tray. The pathologist took it to the lab for a frozen section. In the OR animation was largely suspended. Eliopoulos took two temporary stitches in the incision on Joan's breast to close it. He was the only man in the room.

It is always, Helen Walsh thought, *a kind of sisterly experi-ence on a breast biopsy.* There was a real sense of rooting for the patient.

The circulating nurse said, "What do you think?"

Eliopoulos shook his head. "We'll wait for the pathologist."

As the biopsy stretched out, the tension built. Five minutes is sufficient for a frozen section. It was already seven. The longer the wait the more probable the cancer.

In nine minutes the pathologist was back. He spoke to Eliopoulos at the door. Eliopoulos turned to Helen and the nurses
and shook his head. "Positive," he said. "We'll take the breast."

One of the nurses said, "Shit."

They began all over. A new set of instruments was laid out
by the scrub nurse. A second surgeon, standing by to assist, was
paged. Another scrub nurse came in. They removed all of the
wrappings from Joan's inert form and put new ones in their
place.

Helen Walsh gave Joan a shot of Anectine through the IV
tube. It paralyzed her for about three minutes. She then put a
tube down Joan's throat. At the end of the tube was a kind of
balloon which could be inflated, so Helen could control Joan's
breathing. Helen was now completely responsible for Joan's
life maintenance. Eliopoulos looked at Helen. Helen nodded.
Eliopoulos made a neat careful incision with the skin knife on
either side of the breast, cutting toward the center. Then with
a new knife he began slowly to cut away a little at a time the
subcutaneous tissue. One of the scrub nurses held the skin back
with retractors. Anything suspicious was sent to pathology for
a frozen section. As he cut he tried to avoid as much as possible
the muscle tissue. Periodically the other nurse cleaned out the
surgical area as blood collected. She used a clear plastic tube
with a stainless steel tip like a pencil which vacuumed any area
at which it was pointed. As they went on, the assisting surgeon
cauterized small blood vessels and sutured the larger ones. As
he cut, Eliopoulos was careful to take some lymph nodes for
pathology.

There was no talk now, merely the sounds of the work and
the humming of the life-support and gas systems behind Helen
and of the exhaust fans above. The moving blip of Joan's heartbeat displayed on a scope was a steady punctuation.

The breast came out finally, in one piece, and went to pathology. The skin was folded carefully back in place and Eliopoulos began to stitch. As he did so the second surgeon inserted the drain. Eliopoulos stitched carefully in small tight stitches, his large hands steady and clever as he moved. When he finished, a large pressure bandage went over the incision, the drapings began to come off, and Helen began to wake Joan up.

First she turned down the halothane dosage, then turned off the nitrous oxide. In about five minutes Joan began to stir. Helen removed the tube from her throat and administered pure oxygen. One of the nurses removed the EKG monitor. Another removed the blood-pressure cuff. Helen wheeled her out of the OR and into the recovery room, staying always near her head, ready to turn her if she vomited. In the recovery room Joan's records were handed to the recovery room nurse.

"Her name's Joan," Helen said. "She's had a modified radical mastectomy of the left breast. She expected it, I think, and was pretty well acclimated. I don't think it will be a big shock when she comes to."

For Joan the recovery room was fragmented and barely real. Helen Walsh was there. A nurse was there as well. Maybe Eliopoulos. Was he there? She didn't know. Then Judy Marsh, and she realized she was in her room. She could not remember asking and being told, but she knew with her first coherent consciousness that her breast was gone. *Hello, Jude.* "Hello, Jude." She felt the bandages on her left side. No great mounds of swaddled wrappings, just some gauze and some adhesive. The bandage extended over the breast area and around under her arm. It was not a very impressive bandage. She remembered Dan and his appendectomy and how insignificant a bandage he had come up from surgery with. She drifted in and out of sleep.

"Jude," she said. "You know what?"

"What, Joan?"

She slept. She woke.

"Jude, is that you, Jude?" You know what?"

"What, Joan?"

She went back to sleep. During one moment of awakeness she heard Judy say, "I'm going down and get your chart and see what the medication schedule is. I'll be right back."

"Okay, Jude. Take your time. I'm fine." As she drifted off again she was like a drunk trying to be sober, trying to speak lucidly and intelligently and no one should know that she was zonked. The phone rang. *Isn't it good I got a phone,* she thought. *I can call anyone, and they can call me. But they aren't supposed to call in now. I don't think. I think the switchboard is supposed to intercept after surgery. Hello.* "Hello?"

"Joan? This is Judy."

"Bullshit, Judy just went down the hall. Who is this?"

"Judy Martin, Joan."

"Well who the fuck is it, Judy Marsh or Judy Martin?"

"Joan, it's Judy Martin. From Endicott. How was your surgery? Did they have to take the breast?"

"Yep. The bastards took it."

"Oh, Joan, I'm sorry . . ." Joan let the phone drop and went to sleep. Judy Marsh came back to find it dangling at the end of its cord, humming its high-pitched warning. She hung it up. Joan never remembered the conversation. When she learned that Judy Martin had called in and that she, Joan, had used foul language, she was appalled. Judy Martin would never tell her what she'd said, but Joan knew no one less ready to admire the richness of her foul mouth than Judy Martin.

Judy Marsh sat and watched her sleep, on her back. The IV was still attached to her left hand, the needle in the vein.

Joan woke up. "And she drinks like a fish, Jude. A goddamned fish."

"Who?"

Joan slept again.

A half hour after she was up from surgery Ace came in. He came through the half-open door, walking quietly. Unsure of what he would see. Joan was asleep, Judy was there, small and blond in her white uniform.

"How is she?" he said, softly.

"In and out. She's asleep for a while and then awake, and asleep. There's no pain."

"She know she lost the breast?"

"Oh, yes. She's been awake. She knows."

He stood silently at the foot of the bed, looking at her. Above him high on the wall the television was on, but the sound was down.

"I'll stay a while with her, in case she wakes up," he said. "If you want to take a break or anything."

"Okay. She's not going to be awake very long and very coherently today. She's very foolish. Ten minutes ago she woke up and said, 'She drinks like a goddamned fish' and went back to sleep."

"When David was born," he said, looking at Joan as he talked, "she was scared and had a lot of anesthesia and I came to see her right after the doctor called. I went in, twenty-six years old, the new father, and she was lying there on her back like that with her eyes closed. And I said, 'How are you feeling?' and she opened her eyes and looked at me and said 'Lousy' and rolled over and went to sleep. And I stood around with my thumb in my ear for about twenty minutes and went out and got myself some fried shrimp at Dill's. And many beers."

"I'll leave you for a few minutes," Judy said.

And she left him alone in the room. He felt her loss. He felt nervous without her. *Christ,* he thought, *she's so small you could mail her first class for thirteen cents, and I'm scared when she leaves me alone.* He looked at his wife. *She looks just the same as she always does when she sleeps.* She had on lipstick. He wondered if she'd left it on during the surgery or put it on afterward. *Probably the first thing she did when she woke up.* With the hospital johnny on she looked no different. He couldn't see any meaningful bandages. She looked as she had yesterday. She woke up briefly and they spoke. She went back to sleep and still he stood looking at her. He felt the strong craving in his chest and arms. He wanted to lie on the bed with her and put his arms around her. But he knew he should not. Yet.

In a while, Judy came back in and he went home.

Chapter 17 ⌒

SEVERAL TIMES he called the hospital and Judy told him Joan was still asleep. Shortly before the boys came home from school, he called again and Joan was awake.

"How long I don't know," Judy said. "But why don't you bring them down as soon as they come home. She's lucid enough when she's awake."

It was nearly three when he drove with his sons to the hospital. When they had gone to school he had not yet known if Joan had in fact had a mastectomy. Now, after school, on the short drive to the hospital was the first chance he had to tell them. There was no easy way. Both boys were in the front seat with him.

"Mom is fine," he said. "But she had her left breast removed."

Dan said, "She did?"

David was silent.

"The cyst was cancerous, and they had to take the breast."

"Did you know they were going to?" David asked.

"No, we thought they might, but we felt you shouldn't have to deal with the possibility, only with the fact."

Dan said, "Have you seen her?"

"Yes."

"Does she look funny?"

"No, you can't tell really. There are bandages, but they don't show and your mother has never been known as Barbara Bosoom."

David said, "Has the cancer spread?"

"No. They took tests Monday and Tuesday, body scans."

Dan interrupted, "What's a body scan?"

"X-rays of various parts of her body. X-rays of her bones, liver, lungs, that sort of thing. Anyway the tests all came out negative. That is, there is no cancer in other parts of her body."

"So she's going to be okay."

"Yes." He wasn't as sure as he sounded. "Probably. There's a couple of other tests they will take. But everything looks good." The details of lymph-node involvement and its implications were more than he thought he should ask them to deal with. If there was involvement they would have to deal with it, as he would. If there were not, there was no point in anticipatory fear. He could spare them that. If it were bad they would have the chance to be afraid and to sample the full measure of its badness. But not until they had to, and unless they had to. And what he had answered was true. *It will make my fear no less if they are afraid too. It is not their job to help me deal with fear. That is my job.* John Waynesque phrases resonated inside him that spring. He was aware that they were trite, but they were there, inside him, and he found that in extremes they were true, and they worked. *There are things a man must do* served much better than *woe is me.*

"Can we tell people?" Dan said.

"Mom still has some impulse to keep this a secret, but I think that she will change her mind. It can't be kept a secret. I see no reason why it should be. I think she has a right to require us to be secret until she does change her mind. As far as I'm concerned you can tell everyone you want to anything you want. Will either of you be embarrassed?"

"No."

"No, why should we be embarrassed?"

"No reason, I simply asked. Sometimes a kid might find it embarrassing to talk about his mother's boob. I don't think you would be, but I thought I'd better check."

They seemed sincerely puzzled at the prospect of embarrassment and he was relieved. At least that's not a problem, he thought.

They wheeled into the parking lot at Union Hospital and went up to Joan's room. The boys seemed okay. The loss of a breast didn't seem to hit them much differently from, say, the loss of an appendix. *I wonder, if they were girls would it strike them more? Or is it striking them more than they show? I always tell them to let their emotions out, to express them, let them show. But I always repress mine, and then tend, I think, to learn more from what I do than what I say.* He laughed at himself. *Christ, Bob, you are a profound bastard. You really know kids.*

When they went in the room Dan was frightened. He was scared to see Joan, for fear of how she'd look. When he saw her he thought she looked awful. Lying in the white bed, the IV in her hand, the white bedding rumpled around her. Her lipsticked mouth a bright slash against her white face. *Why did he tell us right before we came?* Dan thought. *She looks awful.*

"Hi, Ma," he said.

She was awake and animated. She seemed completely lucid now. They all knew that she would put out her best for the kids when they came, but even so it was convincing.

"Did Daddy tell you what the operation was?"

"Yes."

"Well, easy come, easy go."

"Besides," Ace said, "now you can get bras at half price."
Once you got an act that works, he thought, *you may as well
keep playing it. Now is not the time to break in new material.*

They already knew, between them in the soundless communication that had evolved out of twenty years together, that this
was the handle they were going to grasp. They had already
established, without once saying so, the basic joke, and they
would work variations on it as long as there was need.

The boys' visit was blurry to Joan. Later they all discovered
that she forgot much during the April days that followed surgery.
She was always lucid and rational when she spoke, but she sometimes repeated things and she forgot things.

On Thursday, April 24, when they went to visit, she did not
know whether they had been there Wednesday. She had a
sense of Ace's presence. Not so much a memory of his visit but
an instinct that he had been there. But she always knew the
breast was gone. It was as if she had never discovered it, simply
that she had awakened knowing it. The way you know that you
have a nose, or that you breathe. It was simply a part of her consciousness.

She felt all right. Wednesday night, after visiting hours, she
had felt some little nausea. She had mentioned it to a nurse, and
almost at once there was a small shot in the buttocks and the
nausea was gone. It never came back.

Ace came right after the boys went to school. She was awake
when he came in and sitting up.

"How is it?" he said.

"Fine, really, I feel okay. The incision isn't bad at all. But
my goddamned left arm hurts like hell."

"That's dumb," he said. "They did not remove your arm,
they removed your boob. Your boob is supposed to hurt."

"Well, it doesn't."

"You can't do anything right," he said.

"Did you cover my class yesterday?"

"Of course not. I stayed home and waited for Eliopoulos to call."

"Did you let them know?"

"I canceled it Monday."

"Jesus, they won't like that."

"They should feel free to discuss it with me when I go in Friday."

"Don't get mad at anyone. Please, I don't want that. I have to work there."

"Me, Mr. Warm?"

"Yes."

"Oh for crissake, Joan. I'm not a goddamned animal. Of course I'll be pleasant. What do you think I am?"

"I know what you are, and I know sometimes if you get mad you can be really lousy to people. And it would just make it harder for me if you blow up at any of the people down there."

"How about I give the whole administration an hour to get out of Beverly?"

"Besides," she said, "I like some of those people."

"Jesus Christ," he said.

"How are the boys?"

"Good, they're okay. They seemed not too shook about it."

"Were they here yesterday?"

"Yep. You talked to them terrific. You were good."

"Good. When are you going to do David's birthday?"

"Today. I got the tickets and everything. I figure we'll just go ahead and do what we were going to do."

"Yes."

"Have they given you anything for the arm pain?"

"I don't know. It's not bad unless I move a certain way."

"What do they say it is?"

"Oh, they talk about lymph nodes and certain glands being removed. But to me it feels like a pinched nerve. You know. Like a hot needle sticking me if I turn a certain way."

"How about the rest of you. The boob area and such?"

"The discomfort is really very minimal," she said. *What a pleasure to listen to her talk,* he thought. *How come I'm a writer and she's not and she talks beautifully and I don't.* Her expressions were so graceful, and her sentences were so full and complete. She seemed always to know ahead of time exactly what she wanted to say. And yet the language rolled out spontaneous and fresh. *Funny. When she tries to write things it doesn't come out. Speaking and writing appear to be different gifts. Another insight. Mr. Deep.*

"All I can compare it to is a sunburn. I don't mean it burns like a sunburn. The sensation is different. But the level of aggravation is about the same. You know. You go to work or clean the house or drive a car when you have a pretty good sunburn and you say to yourself, 'Oh, this sunburn is really annoying.' It never keeps you from functioning. It's just sort of annoying. And you'll be glad when it's better. You know?"

"Is it tight?"

"A little. They took some tissue and the skin is sort of right against the rib cage. There's no padding, and until that rebuilds it will be sort of tight."

"When you come home we can do a little weight work and build that up," he said. "It's just pectoral muscle and if it's slow coming back we can build it up with some bench presses or flies."

"Oh, flies sounds super."

"I got a fly for you," he said.

"They got me up this morning."

"How was that?"

"Okay. Moving around makes my arm hurt but other than that it was okay."

"Want to get up with me?"

"Not right now. Maybe before you go I'll go to the bath-room."

"You want visitors?"

"Yes. I get tired sometimes, but otherwise I'd like them."

"Want me to tell the students to come?"

"You can tell them they can come if they want to."

"Want me to tell them what happened?"

"No. I will do that. I should. They should hear it from me."

"What time do you have to be at the theater?"

"Matinee begins at two o'clock. I'll get the kids out of school early. I already sent a note. We'll come down here around noon, visit you for an hour and then go into town."

"Are you eating out?"

"Yes. I have dinner reservations at the Ritz."

"I feel bad not being there for Dave's birthday."

"I think it was very selfish of you to have breast cancer on your son's sixteenth birthday."

"I went to the bicentennial Patriot's Day parade though."

"You're not all bad," he said. "Have you seen your incision yet?"

"No. Maybe today. I'm kind of afraid to look. How bad could it be though? The bandage isn't that big. Eliopoulos is very happy with it. He says it's one of the best jobs he's done."

"I like a man that takes pride in his work," Ace said. "I would think that the sooner you looked the better off you'd be. Same for me."

"I don't want you to see it. Not yet anyway."

"I should see it sometime. It's not curiosity. It's simply better to know than not to know."

"Not yet."

"Sure, not yet. But when you can. When you're ready. The thought doesn't appall me. It doesn't excite me either. I mean I'm not a scar freak. I just think it should be like everything else, something that we share. I know you got cut, but it's still our surgery, not just yours. It's been harder on you, but only a little."

"I know. Eunie said today they'd change the bandages and she'll tell me if it's okay to look."

"What do you mean okay?"

"Eunie will look and tell me if it's too yukky for me to look at still."

"Yeah, okay." He felt slightly jealous of Eunie. He wanted to be the one to look first and decide on such matters. But he was also a little relieved. Maybe it was quite yukky. Maybe it was better for Eunie to look first. He also knew that there was a matter of shared femaleness there that he could not violate, even if he wished to, and part of him did.

"I think I'll try walking to the bathroom. You want to stand over here."

She sensed his jealousy, his sense of exclusion. She wanted him to help her now, to let him participate, to feel important. For all the mature strength he had, she knew also there was a lot of small boy in there as well. It would help him if now he took her arm and helped her walk.

He stood by her as she moved very carefully to swing her feet off the bed. "Let me take your arm," she said. "You just stand still and I'll hold on to you, okay."

As she got out of bed her arm had the sharp pain in it for a moment until she was upright. She held his arm and pulled herself upright. He was heavy and thick and easy to lean on. As she moved with him toward the bathroom an object like a canteen bumped against his leg. He could see it hanging from her shoulder. "What the fuck is that?" he said.

"It's a, if you'll pardon the expression, drain."

"Yargh."

"I know. Isn't it gross?"

"There's a tube from the incision?"

"Yes, keeps blood and fluid from collecting."

"Okay, okay. I know all I want about that. Does it hurt?"

"No, not all, I don't even notice it."

With her leaning on his arm and him wheeling the IV apparatus besides her, they moved across the room to the bathroom, where she used the toilet, and then he brought her back.

In bed again she felt tired. As if she had walked a long way at a fast pace, and needed now to rest.

"Eliopoulos been in this morning?"

"Yes, early, I think. I'm very blurry."

"What did he say?"

"Everything's fine. They will have to wait for the lymph node biopsy to come back, but everything else is fine."

"How long for the lymph nodes?"

"Two or three days, they said."

"Naturally that takes us into Saturday and naturally that means not till Monday."

"Maybe Friday."

"Not likely," he said.

"Well, we just have to wait."

"Yep. We've come this far. I guess we can go a little farther."

A nurse came in. She was their age, dark-haired and tall, her uniform very crisp. Joan said, "Ace, have you met my friend Eunie. Eunie, this is my husband."

"Hello."

"Hello, Eunie."

"Your wife is the hit of the floor," Eunie said.

"Laugh a minute," he said.

"She really is. She's a super patient."

"You should see her whine when you're not around, Eunie."

"Not me," Joan said. "A little soldier."

"We've got some things to do," Eunie said. "You'll have to step out for a little while."

"What time is it?" He never wore a watch.

"Eleven-ten," Eunie said. "It'll only take a few minutes. You could go down in the coffee shop."

"No, that's okay, I've got to get my kids anyway. I'll pick them up and come back around noon."

"Okay," Joan said. "Bye."

He gestured goodbye with his hand and went out. Eunie closed the door behind him and he went down the corridor, feeling again vaguely shut out.

Chapter 18 ⌒

JOAN'S LUNCH came at five of twelve and she was just beginning to eat it when Ace and the boys arrived. She knew Ace had
been there less than an hour ago. But she couldn't remember
exactly what they said. The boys had each brought her a get-
well card.

Dan's, illustrated with a series of drawings, said, "Some have
two, some have a hundred, some have none, but we love you
best with just one."

David's displayed a busty and sensuous Jane Russellesque
woman on a gatefold card. When you opened the fold one
breast disappeared. The card said,

> Roses are red,
> So is a ruby,
> We love you best
> With just one boobie.

The cards elated her. She felt a little high. Some of this
perhaps was the waning effects of anesthesia, some was relief that
surgery was over, some was a sense that the family was intact,
the cards were loving and relaxed, and the boys were well. They

would bear no scars, she knew. *But there's something in it for me,* she thought. *It's a burden I won't have to bear. I won't have to scheme and work to see that this surgery doesn't damage them. They are not shaken by it, and I don't have that to deal with. That's fantastic.*

"I have a treat for you too, heart of mine," Ace said. "So that your recovery time is not frittered away on daytime TV and gossip with the nurses, I have some reading matter." He brought from behind his back another stack of movie magazines.

She was thumbing through the magazines talking with the boys as she did. Eunie came to take away Joan's empty tray.

"Eunie, look at the cards the boys made."

Eunie read them and laughed. She had children. She understood why Joan wanted her to see the cards. "That's great," she said. "That's super."

"Where did the flowers come from?" Dan asked. There were several plants and two vases of cut flowers in the room.

"I don't remember," she said. "I don't even remember them arriving."

"I'll look," Dan said.

"Do you remember us being here?" David asked.

"No, were you here yesterday?"

"Yes," Dave said, "and we talked about how you felt and the surgery and everything. You don't remember that?"

"No."

Dan said, "Mom," with exasperation.

"Well, I don't," she said. "The anesthesia makes you forget for a while. Helen Walsh told me that would happen. They had to keep me out for quite a while. And she said a big dose like that produces some loss of memory."

"When David was born," Ace said, "after I left from my first visit, where I stood there and she slept at me, they brought her lunch and she ate it and started eating the raspberry Jello for dessert, and fell asleep and the Jello melted and ran all over the spread."

"I woke up," Joan said, "and saw the red all over the sheets and thought I was hemorrhaging and called the nurse in a big panic."

"Were they mad?" Dan asked.

"No, they laughed at me. I was trying to be so cool and under control. You know, 'I beg your pardon nurse, I really hate to bother you, but I think I may be hemorrhaging here.' "

Dan said, "Here's some flowers from Teddie and Kim."

Ace said, "Are you loving the movie mags?"

"Yes. Do you remember the hairdresser I used to go to who found out I was a college professor and used to save the *Atlantic* and *Saturday Review* for me to read while I was in the chair? Everyone else was reading *Screen Mirror* and I had to read *The New Republic.*"

"Fine journal," Ace said. "I got a good review from them last time out."

"Well, I was dying. I wanted my movie mags."

"Why didn't you tell him you wanted the movie stuff?" David asked.

"I couldn't bear to. He was so proud of having the intellectual stuff for me. I couldn't bear to tell him that I was dying to read about Jackie and Ari and Liz and Dick."

Ace stepped into the hall and looked at the clock. It was one o'clock. *If we don't leave now,* Ace thought, *we won't make the theater.* The boys were aware of the time too. Joan appeared not to notice. Ms. Pike, the head nurse, came in.

"I understand," she said, "that there are some get-well cards here that I should see."

"Oh, Ms. Pike," Joan said, "look at these."

Ms. Pike was a former Army nurse, a strapping woman with hard humorous eyes. As she looked at the cards she laughed silently, with her mouth closed. "I'd like to show these cards to a few other patients," she said. "A lot of these people just go all to pieces after surgery. Not even surgery like yours either."

"Well," Ace said, "we probably ought to get under way."

"Oh, no, not yet." Joan said. "I really feel fine now. You don't have to leave yet."

She had forgotten the theater. All three of them knew that simultaneously. And all three of them knew simultaneously that they were not going to say anything. That they were going to stay with her and talk and not mention the theater. None of them said it, but all of them knew that the others knew and there was an unspoken unsignified agreement that they would stay with her as long as she wanted them. And they did.

Dan read off the names of the flower contributors. And they commented on them, not always favorably. Nurses came in and out, to look at the cards that Dave and Dan had made.

At two-fifteen Joan said, "Hadn't you better be getting into Boston. You don't want to miss the play."

"Yeah," he said, "you're right." Neither boy mentioned that the play had been under way already for fifteen minutes."

As they left he said, "We're having dinner at the Ritz, and by the time we get back it will be too late to visit. I won't see you till after your rotten class tomorrow."

"Okay. Have a nice time. I'm sorry I can't go."

"You and me both."

"Have a nice time at the theater, you guys," she said.

"Okay."

"Maybe tomorrow," Ace said to her, leaning back in the door, "when I come tomorrow maybe we'll know something."

She nodded. They left. She wished he hadn't said that. She

had almost been able in the aftermath of surgery to forget the suspended lab report. Until they knew about lymph nodes they still didn't know how bad it was. They still didn't know if she was going to die. He'd been good. He had been, indeed a redwood tree where her fears had nested. But she wished he hadn't shown his apprehension about the lymph nodes.

After surgery was much better than she'd feared. The pain was not anything like she'd feared it would be. In fact much less than the pain of childbirth. At worst there was discomfort. She didn't feel mutilated. The bandages did not look ominous. The reality was so much less unpleasant than the anticipation that her postsurgical mood was up, and she had managed to smother the fear of metastasis.

One more thing. The lab report on the lymph nodes. Then it would be over, everything would be known. Or would it? Would it be that the lymphatic system was involved and there would have to be chemotherapy and radiation and maybe her hair would fall out. And wouldn't it be just as uncertain. *'Now, Mrs. Parker, we can't say for sure. We hope it's arrested. We'll just have to take it a step at a time.' God help me. I wish he hadn't reminded me of the lymph nodes.*

Ace and the boys drove into Boston. It was too late for the theater, but they could stop off at his office, kill a little time there, check his mail, and go to dinner at six when the Ritz opened its dining room doors.

"She didn't seem to know the time," Dave said.

"I know it," Dan said, "and the clock was right there. Why is she like that?"

"I assume it's the aftereffects of anesthesia," Ace said. "This is a heavy dose. Maybe three or four hours' worth, and she's probably getting pain-killers too."

"What are we going to do about the tickets?" Dave asked.

Ace shrugged. "I guess we eat them. I can't go and exchange them after the play is already on, I assume. What we can do is stop at the theater right now and try. If they won't, then I'll just buy some for another time."

As he drove into Boston the thought of waiting until Friday and perhaps Monday for the lab results pressed against his consciousness. To the boys the worst was over and he wanted them to stay that way. To him the worst might lie ahead. *If only there was some goddamned closure. If only there was a point at which someone would say, 'Okay that's it. It's over.' It was the worry, the uncertainty, the dread that busts your balls.* He felt tired, the evening looked very long to him, as he drove automatically through the city. He'd spent so much of his life in it, he drove in it the way he walked in his yard.

He left the station wagon running at the curb on Tremont in front of the Shubert and went into the lobby and bought tickets for another performance. He was embarrassed to ask about exchanging the tickets and he was tired. There was enough he had to make himself do without making himself do this. *Sixty bucks,* he thought. *Sixty bucks won't make much difference to me this time next year, whether I spend it or save it.* But he was embarrassed by his reticence, and the sense he had that it was a weakness. And he told the boys that the theater would not exchange them.

Chapter 19 ⌒

JOAN LAY on the bed after they left and read *Movie Screen Mirror*. *What drivel,* she thought. *I love it.* She read and drifted into sleep and woke and read and the adventures of Dick and Liz merged with her sleep and she wasn't clear if she read about them or dreamed about them. Then Liz gave way to Helen Walsh and Joan was awake again.

"Hi, Helen."

"Joan, I have good news for you," Helen said. Other women were crowding in behind her. "We got the lab report back on the lymph nodes. There's no involvement. It's all negative. There's no lymph node involvement at all."

We weren't supposed to know till Friday, Joan thought. The other women were in the room now. An army of women, it seemed to Joan. Laughing and hugging her and kissing her and hugging and kissing each other. Operating-room nurses, floor nurses, candy stripers, technicians, therapists. The female voices filled with pleasure, women's laughter, excited and very glad, an emanation of tears long retained, now joyfully flowing, these things seemed to flood through her, seemed somehow the exterior manifestation of the posture of her own spirit. She had escaped. She was coming back.

"Oh, Helen," she said.

Helen Walsh nodded, her eyes very bright. "I know," she said, "I know."

Joan wanted to hug them all, everyone who had been there with her, who had cared enough to cry with relief. Who now capered and whooped like Girl Scouts at a jamboree, unencumbered at this moment by men, unformed by the attitudes of husband or father, it was a moment of pure femaleness, of sisterhood much more profound and enveloping than genetic sisterhood could be. It was not a time for Ace or the boys or Benny, the respiration therapist, or Dr. Eliopoulos or Dr. Barry. It was we girls writ large. It was at this brief place their triumph. A triumph that no man could fully share. *My God,* Joan thought, *I am a super broad. So are we all, all super broads.* The euphoria was like something she'd felt before. After the babies were born she had had this same sense of personal and feminine triumph. She could still remember that feeling and she reveled in this one. *By Christ,* she thought, *I have done a hell of a thing. I have produced two magnificent babies and I am a goddamned woman and a half. No one could have done it better.* And the two achievements fused in her mind now. She never knew why exactly that community of sisterhood, and the fusion of childbirth and her own resurrection were so powerful. She was conscious of a great euphoric belonging and a sense of triumph shared with other women.

At bottom, in the pool of their collective unconscious, they all perhaps were gleeful in the ultimate feminine triumph, the life-bearing female victory over death. It was several minutes before she thought of Ace or the boys.

In Boston, Dave and Dan waited in his small square office decorated with David's sketches, photographs of the boys, and a large round bird that Dan had colored in grammar school.

"I'm going to find Gary," he said to them. "Kill a few minutes here while I do." Often they would complain; Dan would say, I want to come too. But now they didn't. It was as if they knew that their father had all he could handle. Looking back at the time later, he couldn't remember them fighting, and they seemed more willing to do what he asked than was their custom. Down the beige hall, the old brick painted new beige, through the hollow-core swinging doors, Gary's office was just like his, but windowless. "Seniority," he always said to Gary. "I'm a big-deal Associate Professor. You are a pishika Assistant Professor. You're lucky they give you a roof over your head."

Gary was in. "Big Bobbo," he said as Ace came through the door. "How is your sabbatical?"

"It sucks," Ace said. "I'm going to tell you some stuff. Then I'm going to ask a favor."

"Okay." Gary was ten years younger, with a modish Caucasian Afro. He dressed carefully and currently. "What's wrong?"

"There is no proper way to react to what I'm going to tell you. I know that. You don't have to worry about how to act.

"We discovered a week ago that Joan had breast cancer, and her left breast was removed yesterday morning. As far as we know she's fine. We'll wait for final biopsy reports tomorrow or Monday."

Gary said, "Jesus Christ."

"I know," Ace said. "She's doing fine. So am I. The thing is, it's David's birthday, and we are going to the Ritz for dinner. I need another adult."

"Sure," Garry said. "Of course. What time are you going?"

"Reservations are for six. I'm just killing time till then."

"Jesus Christ," Gary said.

"I wouldn't have anything to say either. Don't try. We'll just go along like we always do. I'll be Leo Gorcey, you be Huntz Hall."

"Oh, swell," Gary said. "Do I have to pay for dinner too?"

"If you paid for dinner we'd end up at Ugi's famous onion Sub Shop. I'll pay, for my kids' sake. How do you think they feel having dinner at the Ritz with an Armenian?" The banter was as it always was in their friendship, but it was not easy this time for ither of them.

"Why don't you go home and change," Ace said. "And I'll get the kids and pick you up at your place."

"Aren't you going to dress up?"

"I am dressed, turkey."

"But for what?"

"Try not to look like the lead singer in a rock group, okay. This is your basic Ritz."

Gary left and Ace went back down the hall to his office.

Dan was typing and Dave was looking at the books.

"Gary's going to join us tonight, okay?"

Dave nodded. Dan said, "Yes." They both liked Gary. He was ten years nearer their age and very open and easy.

Dan picked up the phone and said, "Let's call Mom."

His impulse was to say no, impatiently. But he knew Dan needed reassurance and he knew there wasn't much to do till six, and he knew Dan would like the idea of calling his mother in a hospital room from his father's office. He could remember himself wanting to do things like that. It was the differentness of it. "Yeah, sure, go ahead. You dial nine, then the number. Here I'll write it down for you."

While Dan dialed he went to check his mail. There was a notice that someone had been named Director of Placement and someone else Supervisor, Buildings and Grounds. There was a flyer from a publisher that proffered a new book to solve the students' writing problems, and there was a short round mailing tube from his London publisher containing advance copy of their dust-jacket design for the English edition of his new novel.

"Hey, Ive," he said to the department secretary. "How's that grab you?" He showed her the jacket. She was a handsome girl with dark hair and black eyes and a mobile face. She twisted the face into a gesture of noncommittal. He turned the jacket over and showed her his picture on the back. It was the same picture that was always used. One of the running jokes among his friends was about how sick everyone was of his picture. "Okay," he said, "how's that one grab you, Cookie?"

She said, "Did you know that you are the same age as my mother?"

"Oh," he said. "That's how it grabs you." They both laughed. *She doesn't know,* he thought. *That's a kind of dividing line in my life. Those who know and those who don't.*

Dan came through the lounge and into the main office where his father was talking to Ivy. "Dad, Mom wants to talk with you."

Ivy said, "Hi, Daniel."

Dan said, "Hi." As Ace went back to his office he could hear Daniel talking to Ivy. *He loves that. He loves adults and being in with them. He's really quite charming sometimes, too.*

When he went into his office Dave was sitting at his desk, drawing on a lined pad he'd found. The phone, off the hook, lay on the desk. He picked it up without disturbing David and spoke standing. He dropped his voice very deep and said, like a ham actor, "Yes, my dear?"

Joan's voice on the other end said, "No nodes."

Daniel had come back in his office too. Ace was very aware of the boys there. They hadn't known of the degree of danger. He shouldn't overreact now.

He said, "None?"

"None. Zero node involvement." A picture of himself at the Ritz eating well. A sense of having sighed very deeply, a sense almost detumescent. How fine it was that Dan had called.

He let his breath out audibly in a long slow sound. "That is a very good thing," he said.

"No chemotherapy. No radiation. Isn't it wonderful?"

"Yes. The boys are right here."

"And you can't talk," she said.

"That's right, but if I could you know what I would say."

"Yes."

"We have here, I think, the light at the end of the tunnel," he said.

"Yes."

"I'll be in tomorrow morning after class, to see you. We'll speak of this then."

"Yes."

"Love," he said.

"Love."

Chapter 20 ~

THAT'S ANOTHER ONE, he thought as he hung up. He had a kind of mental hall of fame where he collected great moments in his life.

"What did Mom want?" Dan asked.

There was when Joan agreed to marry me, and when I came home from Korea, and when we were married, and when the boys were born, and when the first novel was published. And now there's this.

Dan said, "Dad?"

"Mom just wanted to tell me that her last tests came back negative."

Dave looked up from his drawing.

"What's that mean?"

Ace felt a physical effort at control. He had a wordless sense that to overplay his relief would scare them retrospectively.

"It means that the cancer hasn't spread anywhere."

"So she'll be all right," David said.

"Yes, as good as ever, except a few ounces lighter."

"When will she come home?" Dan asked.

"I don't know yet. Next week sometime, I imagine."

"Were you worried about the cancer spreading?" David asked. *He doesn't miss a lot,* Ace thought. *Both of them are more aware than they've let themselves show.*

"I'm glad the tests were negative," he said. "There will be some time in here when Mom may be kind of depressed."

"Why? She's all right now, isn't she?" David said.

"David, she lost a boob, you know," Dan said. He was angry.

"So what. No one can tell."

"Oh, David . . ."

"Okay, don't argue about it, for crissake. Just listen to me for a minute. For a woman to lose a breast is like, well, there is no masculine equivalent. A breast is largely ornamental if you don't breast-feed. But it is part of a woman's sense of who and what she is."

"What's that mean?" Dan asked.

"When a woman is a little kid, she thinks of growing up and becoming a woman. One of the symbols of that is when she begins to get boobs. Boobs tend to make her feel adult and womanly, the object of sexual affection."

"Yes, but you don't care, do you? She's no less sexy to you, is she?" David said.

Jesus, this is tough. "No, but she fears that she might be, and might be less sexy to other men."

"But she's not going to screw with other men," Dan said.

"You bet your ass she's not. But that doesn't matter. She needs to think of herself as sexually desirable, maybe the way I need to think of myself as strong. If something happened somehow and I had to be weak. Maybe that's an analogy. It's not that I need the physical strength all that much. It helps a little maybe when I do carpentry, or for picking up one end of something. But mostly it's ego and sense of self. And it helps fill my shirt sleeves out."

"But she's not a woman because she has two boobs," David said, "anymore than you're a man because you have big muscles."

"That's true. That's logically so. But logic matters less than feeling, and feeling is what we've got here. I think she'll deal with this fine. But I'm telling you it is going to be something she'll have to deal with."

Neither of them looked persuaded. "Take my word for it," he said. *The refuge of parents. Take my word for it. They'll take my word for things about as often as I took my parents' word for things.*

Joan hung up the phone and lay back in the bed, alone now. *It is the light at the end of the tunnel. We won. We beat it. I know I had no control over the fact that the cancer didn't spread. But I feel like I did. I feel like somehow I was a good kid and didn't bitch a lot. I know that's nonsense. I'm just delighted with myself. Okay, I'm going to show them. I can deal with a mastectomy. A mastectomy, that's nothing. Boy am I lucky and am I gonna show them. I'm not sure who them is. The world. Or God who I'm not sure is there. Or the doctors, or I don't know. But I'm gonna show them. Okay, they dealt me this hand with a mastectomy in it. Can I take that? Yes. But the other, the involvement with the rest of the bod. I'm not so sure I could have taken that well. But for now at least I don't have to. So now they're going to see something that will make Betty Ford and Happy Rockefeller eat their hearts out, because I'm going to be wonderful. No chemotherapy. No radiation. I'm going to do just fine now that I know where I stand.*

She pulled her makeup case from the bedside table and opened it. The inside of the cover was a mirror and she held it up away from her to look at her chest. She had her robe on, zippered up and she didn't unzip it. She had no desire yet to unzip it. The bandages made a slightly rounded effect on the left side under the robe and balanced quite equally with the right side of her chest. *Well, if someone comes to visit me they'll barely be able to tell which side is which. The boob that's left is hardly different from the small lump the bandages make. Not being heavily endowed has its advantages.*

The news of her escape changed Joan's entire impulse. Until then she had wanted secrecy. She had wanted to avoid the weight of her cancer and her surgery falling on another person, making them awkward and discomforted. She had dreaded people meeting her and looking surreptitiously and asking themselves, "Which side is it?" Or having her friends think, "Oh, here comes Joan, we'd better be careful what we say."

Now I don't much give a shit about that. I feel so exhilarated. I'm going to feel so good as I recover from this surgery, and the surgery isn't that bad. She wanted to get hold of the feelings. She wanted to be on top of them and keep the feeling of positiveness and strength that she felt now.

I owe somebody something for this. I have gotten a great gift and I owe for it. I wonder whom I want to pay? God, in whom I don't believe? Fate? Mother Nature? I don't know. And it doesn't matter. I need to repay.

'Listen,' she could say, 'it isn't that bad, or at least it wasn't for me. Chances of your developing breast cancer are one in fifteen. But you can catch it early. There are ways. You can examine your breasts. You must learn to do that.' In her mind she was standing before them. All the women. Lecturing. And she realized that the image was from her classroom. She had a special opportunity, she knew. In touch, as she was daily, with young women, at an all-woman's college. 'You must learn to examine your own breasts. And you must do it regularly. You must have a regular checkup and you must demand breast examination.' The classroom was enormous and all the women gazed at her and listened intently. *'And you must remember if it should happen that you knew someone who had it and she was okay. How scary can it be? You should say to yourself, "Look at Joan Parker. She handled it wonderfully." '* She could almost hear the applause, swelling, sustained, heartfelt. She felt good. She could make her contribution. She could have her impact. The idea that the force of her personality could influence others was a very seductive idea. It had always been seductive to her. It was always the source of her greatest self-satisfaction to touch someone's life through the force of her feeling and personality, and to make that life different because of the contact. *I love to be able to do that,* she thought. *That is just the biggest ego trip for me and I have a chance to do this now.*

High-ceilinged and thick with servants, the dining room at the Ritz-Carlton Hotel looked out over the Public Garden, and the lights of cars on Arlington Street. Gary was a good talker and the boys liked him. Ace was able to regroup, as he thought of it, as the meal progressed. He always ate and drank with pleasure and attention, but tonight he was unaware of much that he ate. He thought of something that Winston Churchill had said, *'Nothing in life is so exhilarating as to be shot at without result.'* The phrase stayed in his mind. It lingered in the background of his thoughts and feelings, like background music. He and Gary split a bottle of wine. David wore a pale green leisure suit. Dan had on a double-breasted blazer, light blue with brass buttons. *That suit's getting small for Dave. Shot at without result. Goddamn.*

"Where'd you eat in London?" Gary was asking.

"We ate at Simpson's," Dave answered.

"And lunch at the London Zoo," Dan said. "Yuk."

There was a bottle of Rhine wine in the bucket by the table and one of the waiters poured a bit more in his glass. *When she's out I'll bring her here. Just the two of us. And we'll have any-thing we want and a bottle of wine and maybe two. And we can walk in the Public Garden in the early evening. Before the mug-gers get active.* He smiled inside at his own sense of dispropor-tion, as if he'd shared it with her. He realized suddenly that it was the first time he'd thought about doing something in the fu-ture since she'd gotten sick. *'It better be a big mugger,'* he said to her inside, and laughed out loud inside. *That's one aspect of the excitement. I can start thinking ahead, again. I can plan. I don't have to focus entirely on this day and repel anticipation.* He felt orderly again, but very inward. *'After great pain, a formal feeling comes.'* *It's not what Emily Dickinson meant, but the phrase is good.* The voices of his sons and his friend seemed to come from outside; there was an echo to them. The check came and he paid it and they drove Gary home to Belmont through the new-darkened April night. The car emphasized the containment and new structure of his resurrected life. He looked at Daniel's pro-file beside him as they drove, lit by the city and the dashboard lights. Dan looked just like him. Even he could see it. It was like looking back at himself sometimes. *There I am starting over.*

They got home too late for the hospital and the boys went to bed. He sat alone for a while at the kitchen counter and drank two cans of beer and thought barely at all. He looked very care-fully at the workmanship in the kitchen. At the beams he'd in-stalled in the ceiling, at the stained-glass window in the brick wall. His eye traced the miter line on the molding that framed the window, and he traced along the squared corners of the cab-inets that he'd built. He could still feel the contour of the saw handle and the balance of the hammer in his hand. Things fitted smoothly. There were flaws, but they were hidden and the con-struct was a balanced and serviceable one. The lines were straight. The room was clean. *And well-lighted,* he thought.

And it heals stronger at the break, and all that stuff. Me and you, Ern. He could let himself drink a little now. He could get drunk now. He didn't need to be sure of his control. So necessary had it been that it occurred to him now that he hadn't even wanted to drink. So compelling was the need for holding the center intact that he had instinctively avoided anything that would relax his will. *Well, we've established that. When it gets bad I won't turn to drink, as they say.* He looked at the dog. The dog looked back with that slightly apprehensive alertness he always showed if you stared at him. "I'm okay, kid," he said aloud to the dog. "We're all okay. You too." His voice seemed normal and pleasant to him. It was at home in the room. He felt comfortable talking aloud to the dog. It was as close as he would come to praying.

Chapter 21 ⟿

THE IV came out. Eunie removed it. Another bond loosened. Now she could walk about. Go downstairs, visit Gerry Wilkinson. The IV had never hurt; it was simply like being on a leash. When Dr. Eliopoulos had it removed two days after surgery it was another step, as she put it, "on the old comeback trail, Doctor." He smiled, and opened her johnny to check the incision.

"Have you seen the incision yet?" he asked.

"Not yet."

"You ought to look. It is one of the best things I've every done."

"Gee, that's good to know, Doctor. I'd really hate it if you kept looking at it and shaking your head, and saying, 'How could I have been so clumsy?' That would make me very nervous."

He laughed. "I wouldn't blame you."

Three young girls in uniform stood a little uneasily by the door. Eliopoulos said to Joan, "I've got some student nurses here I'd like to show this to. Okay?"

"Oh, don't worry about me," she said and laid her head back on the pillow and put the back of her hand to her forehead.

The students hesitated. Eunie said, "Go ahead girls, don't pay any attention to her. It's a terrific incision."

The girls crowded around and murmured approvingly.

Joan said, "How about a small round of applause. Let's hear it for the incision."

The girls laughed.

"Lucky they didn't start shouting encore in the operating room. I might have ended up with a bilateral."

Eliopoulos laughed without noise.

"Come on, ladies," he said to the student nurses. "That's enough entertainment. We'll have to look at some other patients."

They left and Eunie began to wheel the IV stand out.

"I think we better look, Eunie," Joan said.

"It's really nothing, Joan," Eunie said. "It's really just a simple little scar, goes across not up and down, and it'll be fine."

"Okay. You look first and tell me if it's okay. If it's fiery red and angry-looking, or puckered or too yukky-looking for me to look at, you say so, and I'll wait."

It was a lot of weight to place on Eunie, but she trusted Eunie entirely, and she knew that Eunie would tell her what was best. Eunie flipped the bandage back and took a long look at the incision.

"Joan, it's really a very good piece of surgery. It's not yukky. Go ahead take a look."

She looked.

Stitches show, that's a little funny. To see thread sticking out of you. But other than that, it's like when I was little. Like the chest was before I reached puberty. Or like a young boy's chest, except that there's no nipple.

"Well," Joan said, "that's not so bad." It was a transverse scar, perhaps seven inches long, running from the sternum to her armpit. The skin was still slightly puckered, and the black thread showed a little. But there was no crater, no gouged and ugly hollow where once her breast had been. Just a small line across her chest and a slight sense of imbalance, because on the right side was nipple and areola, round and central, while on the left was line, straight and extended.

"It's not that one side is flat and the other sticks out," she said to Ace when he arrived after class.

"That's for sure," he said, with the big smile he'd worn since he had stuck his head in the door and grinned at her in speechless delight for nearly a minute.

"It's more that there's a nipple on one side and a line on the other."

"How about under the arm?"

"I asked Eliopoulos that yesterday morning while he examined me. I can't see under there without getting up and looking in the mirror and I haven't felt like that yet."

"What'd he say?"

"He said there's a small depression there which will fill in as soon as the fatty tissue begins to rebuild."

"I've never had any trouble at all regenerating fatty tissue," he said.

"I know," she said. "But the front part, what I can see, is just a little scar. I mean it was sort of an anticlimax when I looked. I'm not sure what I expected exactly, but what I got was . . . just a scar."

" 'He had been to touch the great death,' " Ace said, " 'And after all it was but the great death.' "

"Who said that?"

"Stephen Crane. And me."

"There's something bizarre about being a one-boob person, obviously, but there's nothing repellent."

"When do I get a look?"

"Not yet. The incision is pretty fresh. I'd just as soon give myself every break I can."

"Whatever you say. I'm ready when you are. I don't care whether I see it or not, but, you know, I think it would be better for you when I've looked and not shuddered."

"I know. I want you to see. But not yet."

"It won't make any difference, you know."

"I know. And to you I believe it. I really do. I know it won't make any difference to you, and you don't need to be told how much that helps. But to everybody else it will matter."

"I don't know. I've never discussed it with anyone, and who would tell me the truth now. No one's going to tell me that they can't get it up for a woman with one breast. Unless they didn't know. And letting them say something like that to me and then find out later, that would be lousy. I couldn't do that."

"I know. I'm not asking you. I know that to anyone but you the idea that under my bra is one breast and one falsie . . . I know that it will turn them off."

"Like I said, I don't know. I don't know that it's not true, but I don't know that it is. I could get it up for a one-boobed woman but I'm not unbiased. But other one-boobed women . . . I could lust after them."

"Probably. But because of me you're educated. You love me and lust for me, and would have to lust for others too or admit that I wasn't desirable."

"Yeah, true. So we don't know. We don't know either way."

"But I feel that it's true. Which is about the same thing."

"True. If you had to prove something to yourself I would understand that."

"You mean have an affair?"

"Affair seems a little extended. Let's say, poetically speaking, if you wanted to do it with someone else to prove that you were desirable, I could take that."

"No, I think I can deal with that. I think I can accept the fact that from this point on I will not be viewed as attractive, seductive, appealing . . . whatever. I can do that by having some other things going for me."

"It's not a fact. It's only a possibility."

She gestured that aside with her hand. "You know what I mean. I like to be viewed by men, and women too, as sexy, seductive, intelligent, humorous, articulate; I like people to see me in all those ways. Walking around a one-boobed person, I don't think many people will see me that way."

"Say you're right. I don't necessarily think you are, but say you are. So what?"

"So, not many guys are going to say, 'Hey, I'd like to hop into the sack with her,' and not many women are saying 'Hey, I bet a lot of guys want to hop into the sack with her.' Especially because of what they think is under the bra. If I could show them the scar it would be easier, but remember what you imagined. Maybe you still do."

He shook his head.

"But lots of people will be imagining ugliness under there, mutilation."

He nodded.

"And those people are not going to want to screw me."

"Say you're right. It's not like you are giving up an active extramarital sex life. If it weren't for me you'd still be a virgin."

"If you'd get more than thirteen inches away from me at a party maybe I could have done something about that."

"Thirteen inches was just the right length."

"Hah."

"Never mind Hah. It's a goddamned howitzer."

"Derringer."

"Well, close enough. But the point remains, you don't really want to screw around."

"I know, but I want people to want me to. It has always been my choice. Now it's theirs."

"Yeah, I understand that, of course. You just find yourself in the condition I've been in all my life."

"Despite the howitzer."

"I guess the word wasn't out. Come to think of it neither was the howitzer."

"Well, if I have to rethink myself as a nonseductive person, I can do that. I can substitute taking this well."

"Nobility," he said. "Instead of sexy you can be brave, and a fine example."

"Yes. Even though I am giving up forever being, for lack of a better term, a sex object."

"Except to me."

"Except to you. Even though I'm giving that up forever, I can replace that with some valuable things. I can be perceived as someone who has faced a scary thing and done it bravely, and stylishly. People can admire that. People can be helped by my example."

"Yes," he said.

"People can think 'Wow, she's some lady, look how she dealt with this and overcame it and incorporated it into her life.' "

"I think that some myself," he said. "I also think about slipping into the hospital bed and belaboring you with my howitzer."

"You remember how you said all your life no one considered you a sex object?"

"Yes?" He fed her the straight line, feeling the old delight.

"Well, you were absolutely right, Bob."

"Without exception?"

"Everyone who knows you would agree."

"Absolutely everyone?" He could feel the laughter bubbling up inside. It was a game they had played a thousand times.

"Everyone," she said.

"And you came across for me, why?"

"Pity," she said.

He laughed aloud, the smile that had never left his face expanding into a roar of pleasure.

"You know when I said you could screw somebody else to restore your confidence?"

"Yes." It was her turn with the straight line.

"Well, if you do it's best you choose someone you don't like, because I'm going to kill him afterward."

"Oh Bob," she said. Bob was a code word. She was always kidding when she called him Bob. "You are an understanding person."

"You better believe it," he said.

Chapter 22 ⟿

Saturday, April 26

AND THE VISITORS CAME. *I need this,* Joan thought. *My decision to be brave rather than alluring needs an audience. I need feedback to make it work.* Every visit was, for Joan, a performance. Everyone who came had to be put quickly at ease. *Yes, I lost a couple of ounces of boob over there, but I'm still what I was and you needn't worry.*

Charlotte Tannheimer came. One of the first visitors outside the family. She came into the room with a great rosebush. She was a very small woman and she had brought a very large rosebush and Joan was able to imagine for a moment that the rosebush had brought Charlotte.

She stood at the foot of Joan's bed with the rosebush and she couldn't speak. Tears ran down her face.

"Easy come, easy go, Char," Joan said. "I'm fine and the news is good."

"Oh, Joan," Charlotte said.

"Charlotte, that is the biggest goddamned enormous huge rosebush I've even seen."

"How are you, Joan?"

"Terrific. I'm fine and I feel wonderful about the rest of my life. Now put down that christly grotesque tree and sit in the chair and tell me gossip about Endicott."

Charlotte was all right then. She put the rosebush on the windowsill and sat by the bed and talked with Joan for an hour. The pattern of the visits was established and it would vary little for the remainder of her stay. For Joan it was wearying in some ways, but simultaneously she was center stage and she loved it. The turnout of visitors was an enormous ego booster. She found that people cared about her. She had always known that she had friends, but she had never experienced such an outpouring of affection, particularly female affection. The women cared very deeply.

Sunday, April 27

Eileen Ganem drove up from Plymouth her first day home from New York. She came into the room tentatively, as everyone did the first time, on tiptoe, and burst into tears. They had been friends since before the children.

"Easy come, easy go, Ei," Joan said. "I'm fine, I really am. All the news is good, and I had so little to lose." She did the little patter that had become smoother and more effective with practice. There was no insincerity in it. She meant it each time, but it was a technique she was mastering and it worked. In a few minutes Eileen was all right. *How much she cares,* Joan thought. *Christ, she came in crying. I knew she'd care, but how much, isn't it wonderful how much.* Eileen had brought makeup and nail polish and shampoo. She helped Joan wash her hair, helped her set it. She put nail polish on for Joan, and helped her with the makeup. *I can wear polish. My nails weren't going to turn blue.*

Monday, April 28

Embeth Nagy came and June Crumrine, who had seen them check in and wondered silently why. Eileen took on the chores Ace wasn't good at. She was there almost daily with eye shadow, a new kind of blusher, a new robe. The room filled with flowers and get-well cards. Extra chairs had to be moved in. There was a celebratory atmosphere, a kind of continuing party, in which people came and went, but the music continued.

"It's like a goddamned carnival," Ace said. "How about tomorrow I bring in a couple of six packs and a record player and we have a sock hop." He resented it sometimes. He would have liked a little less company occasionally, but he enjoyed it too. It was fun to go and see who would be visiting and it was fun to watch Joan work. Her color was high, and with company she was very animated. Sitting up in bed, her eyes shiny with excitement, she talked and laughed and gestured elegantly and he watched in a luxury of pleasure. *I could watch her forever,* he thought. *Absolutely forever.*

Nurses came and went. One always seemed to be there. The boys were there afternoons and evenings. They enjoyed the social occasions too. Especially Dan, who was particularly stimulated by grownup conversation. Except for Ace and the boys, most of the men who came seemed a little subdued. They were not apparently bothered by the operation, but they were vaguely out of place. It was a female celebration, a gathering of women, at which men were welcome but not central. Judy Marsh was there. To Joan it seemed she was always there, as if they had done this together. Dr. Barry came in each morning, not simply to look at her chart and smile encouragingly, but to talk. To talk about children and colleges and teaching, about the practice of medicine, about ideas and things that had happened.

Tuesday, April 29

When Ace came in that morning he was the first. Visiting hours had not yet begun.

"You have to get out," Joan said.

"My presence is making you lustful, and you're afraid you won't be able to contain yourself."

"Wrong. The Reach to Recovery lady is coming and she wants to talk with me alone."

"She can't talk in front of me?"

"No. I mean she will probably want to show me her incision and things. It would be awkward for you to be there."

"You're not just making that up because you're ashamed of your libidinous impulses, are you?"

"If they were directed at you I'd be ashamed of them. Now get out for a half hour or so, she's going to be here any minute."

"Balls," he said. There was a small tap on the partially open door. Ace made a face at Joan and opened the door fully. A short plump youngish woman stood there.

Ace said, "Hi, come on in. I'm on my way out."

"Thank you." The woman came in uneasily, as if unsure where to stand.

Ace said, "I'll be back, Snooky," and went out.

"Hi," Joan said. "I'm Joan Parker, won't you sit down."

The Reach to Recovery Program is sponsored by the American Cancer Society. Its goal is to help women to adjust to mastectomy by bringing them into contact with women who have undergone mastectomy. Joan thought it a fine idea. She wanted to talk with someone who had faced mastectomy, who had weathered and coped and triumphed and recovered.

The Reach to Recovery lady sat. She held in her hand some pamphlets. She didn't look at Joan and she seemed to have trouble getting under way. Joan waited a moment and then realized the woman was not going to lead.

"I'm feeling really super," Joan said to her. "There is no node involvement, I feel fine, and I'm not very depressed about losing a breast."

"Gee, that's swell," the Reach to Recovery lady said. "I had mine about five years ago, and it was just awful. I was so depressed."

"Well, I can understand how that could happen," Joan said.

"Would you believe I only weighed a hundred and eight pounds when I went in for my surgery?"

Joan smiled. She couldn't think of anything to say.

"I went into such a depression that I just ate and ate."

"Well, I'm doing fine," Joan said. "My husband and my boys are really supportive, and we're all doing very well so far."

"Wow, that's great. My husband wasn't very supportive. You're really lucky."

"But," Joan said, "you've been able to put that all behind you now. Put your life back together."

"I guess so."

"And this work must be rewarding. Helping people, being able to support them and help them work through their problems."

"Well, I'm still awfully new at it."

"Is that so? You certainly are doing well at it."

Ace sat on a window ledge at the other end of the hall where he could see Joan's door. The Reach to Recovery lady stayed a long time. He whistled "Take the A Train" to himself and played drums on the tops of his thighs. It was a Four Freshmen arrangement he was whistling, and in his head he could hear the Freshmen singing it. He watched one of the nurses walk down the corridor away from him, her skirt tight over her buttocks. *Damn nurses' uniforms simply are not flattering. I think it's the white stockings. Nice ass though. 'The fastest, the quickest way to get to Harlem.' What a great name, Billy Strayhorn. 'You'll get where you're going in a hurry.'* The young nurse with the tight skirt came back down the corridor, walking toward him, her hips swinging. *It's like looking at art. It's not really lecherous, it's merely the pleasures of an aesthetic configuration. I can do it now, I can look lecherously and without obligation at women. I don't have to wonder if soon I'll be looking in earnest. Looking in earnest would suck.*

The Reach to Recovery lady came out and walked down the corridor toward him. He started up the corridor to Joan's room. He smiled at her as they passed. She didn't say anything.

"Oh, the poor thing. She's in much worse shape than I am."

"She's in much worse shape than I am."

"No, I mean emotionally. I was cheering her up."

"She tell you anything about prosthesis?"

"She said she'd go with me when I got out of the hospital and show me the best place to go and help me get fitted. She's really very sweet. But . . ." Joan shrugged. "It's difficult for her. Too bad. The idea is a good one. You know it would be really helpful to any woman to have someone to talk to. I don't need to so much because I have you and everyone is so supportive. The boys are good, and Jude and Eileen and everyone. But for some women, like this poor lady today, it's a shattering and lonely experience."

"You've got you, too," he said.

"Yes, that's true. I know that I have good resources of my own. But it would be much harder if you and the boys were, say, repulsed by the whole thing."

"I didn't marry you for your boobs, babe."

"Anyway, I've got other people to talk with. Mrs. Bacheldor has a friend she says I should talk to who's had a mastectomy, and one of the operating room nurses has had one and maybe I'll talk with her."

"What's Eliopoulos say about Reach to Recovery?"

"I think he has reservations. He doesn't mind them coming around and offering help, but he doesn't want anyone giving me an exercise program but him. He said he doesn't want his terrific incision screwed up."

"I'd listen to him," Ace said.

"Yes, I will. But I am really hot to exercise. I want the full use of the arm and the old bod."

"Me too."

"I thought you would," she said.

"Ask him about weights," Ace said. "Tell him I know something about that and maybe a little light stuff, some light reps would be a good thing when you're ready. If what's missing is pectoral muscle, that may be the easiest muscle in the body to build up. You can do some bench presses and things, if you want."

"I'll mention it to him," she said.

"There's also the full-body press."

"What's that?"

"That's when a two-hundred-and-twenty-pound man lies on top of you and . . ."

"Never mind, Bob."

Chapter 23 ⌒

Wednesday, April 30

AND THE STUDENTS came from Endicott. Sometimes the girls came alone, sometimes they came in groups, three or four at a time. In each instance Joan had to tell them and then relieve the weight of their knowledge, had to be upbeat and easy in her presentation. The girls took it well and responded to the vitality of Joan's recovery.

"And how's Big Bobbo doing in class?" she asked.

"He's just like you said he was," Teddi told her.

"He does not look happy coming into class," Kim said.

Joan laughed. "Oh, you should hear him bitch about it."

"He's nice though," Teddi said.

"Oh, yes," Kim said. "He's nice in class. But you know he is not pleased."

"I am going to ask you ladies," Joan said, "not to tell anyone on campus what my surgery was. I would prefer to tell them myself. When I come back I'll tell my classes. But I would rather they hear it from me."

Both girls nodded and promised. Joan made the request of every student who came to visit. As far as she knew everyone kept her promise. No one told.

And Sharon Taylor came. Joan had not seen her since her abortion and she had a double problem with Sharon. Joan had to tell her of the surgery and relieve her guilt feelings. *I want to rub her nose in it a little too,* Joan thought. *I may be Nora Noble, but I will get a little revenge pleasure too, before I help her through it. But not much. She was a plus. Her dilemma helped us think less about ours.*

"Sharon," she said, "let me tell you about my surgery." It was devastating for Sharon. Her eyes filled and she flushed as Joan told her.

"Oh my God, Mrs. Parker." Joan knew the memory of all their conversations was coming back and painfully, to Sharon. She had said that the Parkers could never know the kind of pain she and Mike were suffering. She had spent hours talking about her problems to a woman who had breast cancer. "Oh my God, Mrs. Parker."

"Sharon. You and Mike were good for us," Joan said. "Your story, weaving in and out of our own, that was a good thing. It was not wrong for you. And it gave us something to do and something to think of. You helped us through this."

"But all the time Mike and I were there, talking about ourselves."

"Ace and I both feel that it was much better than us talking about ourselves," Joan said. "That would have been the pits."

For Joan the students were another reward. She invested a large part of herself in them. And their visits and their concern for her were, as she said, "a payoff. My investment in them has really paid off."

"Ms. Chips," Ace said, alone with her briefly after visiting hours before he went home.

"Look at the cards," she said. "And the flowers. The kids have really rallied round. They care. I needed to know that."

She was high, he knew. Animated as she always was by human feedback.

Thursday, May 1

Ruth Sullivan came to visit. A very tall big-breasted woman, wearing an incongruous wig. She had the soft voice and lack of affect of someone who's had extensive analysis. She taught English with Ace at Northeastern, and she too had breast cancer. Joan was never clear on the details of Ruth's cancer, they were not close friends, but she remembered the visit vividly as one full of unspoken things and inarticulate questions. With Ruth were two other women and the husband of one of them. Ace was there. They never mentioned Ruth's cancer, but Joan sensed that Ruth wished she could. The tension was very tangible beneath the bright chatter. The women seemed less easy than anyone had. Joan knew that among them there were feminist positions more extreme than hers, and she felt a certain disapproval from them at her willingness to undergo mastectomy, and almost a disappointment that it was not a more crucial moment in her life.

When they left Joan said to Ace, "Jesus, there was a lot that wasn't being said."

"Yeah, Ruth really wanted to talk with you, I think, but she couldn't bring herself to it. Maybe if she'd been alone."

"Maybe," Joan said, "she'll call me."

Chapter 24 ⌣

JOHN ELIOPOULOS came to examine her. She was lying in bed, wearing her robe with a guaze pad sewed inside it over the proper spot.

"What the hell is that?" Eliopoulos said, when he pulled the robe back to look at the incision.

"My sister's coming," Joan said.

"My question stands," Eliopoulos said.

"We have given new meaning to the term sibling rivalry, my sister and I. She's coming in from the West Coast tomorrow and when I found that out I sent Eunie and Norah chasing around for padding. She's not going to see me with one boob."

Eliopoulos looked at her incision. "She's not going to see you here," he said. "You look too good. Get the hell out of here."

"Today?"

"Yes. Do you want to stay?"

"No."

"Then beat it."

"How soon can I leave?"

"Right now. Get going."

Nine days after surgery, Joan thought, I'm going home nine days after surgery. She had thought it would be more. It buoyed her that she was going early. I've got to get organized. I've got to pack.

"I'll have one of the nurses come down and remove the drain," Eliopoulos said.

Joan nodded. Her mind was busy with going home. I've got a bra okay, and I can wear my flowered blouse with the beige wrap-around skirt.

Eunie and Norah came in. "Okay, Joan, time for the drain to come out." Eliopoulos was gone. Joan rolled onto her right side and Eunie undid the johnny in the back and let it fall open. She could feel Norah snap off a small piece of tape near her hipbone, on the left side. She'd never really paid much attention to the drain. It had not bothered her. She hadn't really felt it much on the left side. Parts of the left side were still numb. She glanced down to see where it left the incision. It didn't leave the incision. It emerged from her body above and slightly back of her left hip.

"Jesus Christ," she said.

"What is it?" Eunie said.

"Where does that thing go to?"

"Up to the incision."

"But Jesus, it's inside me."

"Yes," Norah said, "didn't you know that?"

"No. You mean you're going to pull that whole long tube down out of my body?"

"It won't hurt," Norah said.

"It really won't," Eunie said.

"I can't stand it," Joan said. "I can't. I've taken everything else, but I can't stand this."

"Joan," Norah said. "I promise it doesn't hurt. It is nothing. Don't look and you won't even know."

"It's got to come out," Eunie said.

Joan shook her head. "It makes me sick to think of it."

"Joan, we haven't told you anything since you came in here that wasn't so," Eunie said. "This is nothing. I'll take hold of your hand and Norah will take out the tube. It will be over in two seconds and it won't hurt a bit. Come on. You've come this far. Once more. Just once."

Joan nodded. Eunie took her hand. Joan pressed her face into the pillow, she felt nauseous. Her whole body clenched in on itself. And as she pressed her eyes tight, the little kaleidoscopic patterns moved in the darkness behind her eyelids.

"Okay," Norah said. "It's done." The nausea settled. They had been right of course. It hadn't hurt. *The big C doesn't let go that easy, does it.*

Ace showed up after class in his normal state of irritation that he had to teach her classes on his sabbatical. It was an irritation intensified by his dislike of the college and modified by his knowledge that it made her happy.

"I'm going home," she said.

"Today?"

"Yes."

"Right now?"

"Yes."

The house is clean. A vision of himself and the boys picking up the house last night appeared in his head. *'It'll take two days to pick up this goddamned armpit,'* he heard himself say to them. *'So we'll start tonight.'* — *'But she won't be home for two or three days'* — *'We'll start tonight anyway.'* And so, with some grumbling, the boys had helped and the house had been put in order. Once begun they had carried beyond getting a start. They had finished. He smiled at the image he carried of Daniel pushing a vacuum cleaner, the handle at eye level, vigorously about his room.

"Let us begin," he said to Joan. "I'll start carrying plants and stuff out to the car."

Joan packed all but the clothes she would wear home. When Ace came back from moving the last of the plants down to the car, Eunie was there helping Joan get dressed.

"Don't look," Joan said from the bathroom.

She had on her skirt and Eunie was helping her put on the bra. She didn't have complete movement in her left arm yet and she had some trouble getting her arm through the strap.

"All right, good, okay." Eunie murmured encouragement. "Now, I've got this gauze here. We'll just stuff in enough to make the sides match."

"That's not going to use up a whole hell of a lot, Eunie," Ace yelled through the half-open door of the bathroom.

"Isn't he awful," Eunie said. "Shut up and carry your plants."

"I've got a Band-Aid here, Eunie, why don't you just peel the gauze off it. That should be enough."

Joan said, "Bob, go in the closet and wait there."

The bra chafed a little. The way it does on a sunburn. Not intolerable, just a little rough feeling. Eunie helped her slip on her blouse. Joan buttoned it up. "Okay, Bob," she said through the door. "Get yourself under control. Here I come."

"Be still my heart," he said. She came out of the bathroom and there she was. The same one he'd brought in. A little slimmer maybe, she'd lost five pounds, but the same one. Her makeup was careful. Her hair was in place. She appeared to have two breasts, and she was resonant with life. *Technicolor,* he thought, *it's like she's technicolor and the rest of the world is black and white.*

She stood still in front of him for a moment, inviting comment.

"Stay close to me on the way out," he said. "In case a passion-crazed intern makes a move on you."

He took the suitcase and she walked ahead of him. She looked fine except that she held her left arm bent a little and close to her side. It took them time to get out of the hospital. There were goodbyes to the nurses, to Benny, to other patients on the floor. It reminded him of when he'd come home from Korea, saying goodbye to people who knew a special thing that you knew, and the joy of deliverance was mixed with the sadness that a special sharing was over. He stood a little aside while she did all of this. He would miss them too. But not the way she would and this was her event.

They said almost nothing on the ride home. There was no need for it, retracing the route they had taken three weeks ago, driving home after driving so often to doctors and to hospitals, driving home with the knowledge that they had, after the knowledge with which they had driven for three weeks, the driving home itself was commentary and celebration. And they knew it. And they didn't need to say so. The celebration was wordless and profound.

They drove up Canterbury Road with the maple trees in early buds. *April's first green is gold,* he thought. For Joan it was a new street. The houses that had stood there since that March day sixteen years ago when she had moved here, thirteen months pregnant as a neighbor had remarked, were different now. The paint was fresher, the shapes sharper against the sky. The maple trees that had stood there since the road had been cut from the Lynn Woods forty years ago, had new grace to the arch of their branches and a new sleekness to the smooth bark on the youngest limbs.

The dog was in the front yard as they drove up. He hadn't seen Joan in three weeks.

"I wonder what he'll do," Joan said. Ace pulled into the driveway and Joan sat for a minute looking at her house. The dog stood poised in the middle of the yard, his gaze fixed on the car, his head tilted slightly to the side. Joan opened her door and got out. The dog raced toward her and past her and jumped into the bacᵏ seat and sat down and looked out the window.

"You got a real way with dogs," Ace said. "We all missed you like that."

Judy Marsh was in Joan's house. *Always,* Joan thought, *always when I need her.*

"I called the hospital and they told me you'd checked out," she said. "I thought I better get over here and see what the house looked like."

"You imply I am a slobbo, Jude?" Ace said.

"He probably thinks the house is clean, Jude," Joan said.

"It is," Ace said. "The boys and I cleaned it last night. It is spotless."

Joan said, "Is it, Jude?"

Judy said, "Ha."

Joan went into the house. Without speaking she went from room to room and stood in each and looked at it. Her husband and her friend stayed outside. *He didn't dust, and he didn't vacuum good. But he picked up, and by his standards it is clean.*

Chapter 25 ~—

RE-ENTRY. The boys came home from school prepared to visit and found their mother home. Eileen Ganem drove up that day from Plymouth to find Joan's hospital room empty, the bed newly made, the flowers gone and no sign of Joan.

"Jesus Christ," she said to Joan when she arrived at Canterbury Road. "I thought the grim reaper had come. I was running around the hospital like a goddamn maniac, asking where you were. I thought you'd cashed in the old chips."

Midafternoon Joan's sister arrived. She was dealing with a difficult divorce and the need to find a job and Joan's experience had hit her hard.

"Chummy's shook about this," Ace said to Joan in the kitchen as he poured a glass of wine.

"She's always been crazy about her boobs," Joan said, "and I suppose she's got to be thinking if it could happen to me it could happen to her."

They sat in the family room and drank wine and talked, and Joan was exhausted and thrilled. Students came, detoured from the hospital, and drank some wine and talked and left, to be replaced by others. Neighbors were there. Ace had to go to Donovan's for another gallon of Gallo Rhine Garten.

Saturday was a day like Friday, with people coming and Joan talking and between visits cleaning her house and feeling the weakness that the three weeks had brought her and reveling in the excitement and the homeness.

Saturday night they sat in the Marshes' kitchen and drank a little beer and wine and ate some raw vegetables with sour cream dip and Joan decided that Monday she'd go back to work.

"The students keep coming and coming. In a way I love it," Joan said, "but they stay so long. I'm better to see them in a more controlled situation. If I am in the classroom I can leave when I want to. Now I can't seem to get them out of my house."

"I can." Ace said.

"Not that way. I love seeing them. I just need to get them out better. Going back to work will take care of that."

"But Ace won't be able to do your classes anymore," John said, "and rap with the students and your fellow professors."

Ace said, "Yarrgh."

And so she would do it. Not four to six weeks after surgery, as Dr. Barry had suggested, but twelve days after surgery. *I am absolutely wonderful. I am going back to work and I'm going to do it in twelve days after a mastectomy.*

Sunday she raked leaves. Her left arm still had a limited range, but she used it as a fulcrum and raked with the right and looked natural. Neighbors questioned if she should work so hard so soon and she loved it.

Monday she went to work. She couldn't drive the car yet, and there was a wordless fear that they both had. She shouldn't be alone yet. They had been afraid too long. They couldn't let go at once. So he drove her and sat in the car in the parking lot and read the *Globe* and drank coffee from a paper cup while she told her classes of her surgery.

When she came into the classroom, its tables undisturbed, its bookshelves and décor exactly as it had been three weeks before, she felt a moment of fierce self-doubt. The inviolate normalcy of the classroom set her back. *What if no one gives a shit?* she thought. *Here I am all primed to tell a drama-laden tearjerker of a story, filled with pathos and power, and what if no one gives a shit about my boob.*

But she was committed and she went ahead. It was difficult to do. The students were obviously glad to see her back. As she began to speak the pleasure went out of their faces and an uncertain apprehension replaced it.

"And so," she said, "I reached up to shave under my left arm and my hand brushed against a lump in my breast."

As she went on several of the girls put their heads down on the desks. Many of the girls had tears in their eyes. The tears and the heads down and the fear in their eyes was difficult for Joan. But she felt she must.

"Some of you will have a lump in your breast," she said. "It probably won't be malignant but you must learn to examine your breasts. You must remember that if it is malignant, it is not the worst thing that can happen. If it happens to you remember that you know someone to whom it happened, and remember how I was back and feeling good twelve days after they took a breast. And remember if they have to take it, it's a lot better than a lot of things. And it is not so ugly a thing."

Thirteen days after surgery she went with him when he spoke at Bradford College. It was dinner first and some drinks and then the speech and no one could tell and she felt good. The bra still rubbed a bit and she got tired quicker, but no one could even guess there was anything wrong and it was an act of pride that she proceed with her life.

Driving home from Bradford she said to him, "I'm going to have some sort of postoperative depression."

"Are you going to start now?"

"No, but it's bound to come," she said. "It's naïve to think it won't."

"It'll be a lot better than the preoperative one we were both in."

"I wonder how I'll handle it."

"You'll handle it as well as you handled everything else," he said. "I'm not so sure it will come at all."

"Oh, I think it probably will," she said. "Like after the babies. There's the old postpartum blues. There will probably be some reaction. You too. You'll need some kind of emotional shakedown."

"Well," he said, "if you get too depressed we can apply the miracle cure, Parker's internationally acclaimed beef injection."

"The thought of that is bringing on my depression," she said.

It was dark and the dashlights of the car softened appearances. The chance to be enclosed with her, surrounded by darkness, excited him. Delimited by the moving car, the privacy of their shared space was romantic to him, and he very carefully patted her thigh. "I'm waiting for physical recovery, sweets, I'm after your body. Screw the postop depression."

But it came. There was no sudden shock, no startling realization. There was a period of more than a week when she had gotten back to work, and the pace of her life had begun to move more normally, that she went over and over the events in her mind. It was in some way deliberate.

I've got to assimilate this experience into my whole life's experience. I have to know what really happened to me. I will make sense of it gradually and not bury it and have a breakdown two months from now.

And so when she was alone she would rerun the events of the past three weeks. She wasn't on stage now, she wasn't putting on a show. Now she was alone and it was time to face a real fact. She was different now: she had but one breast. *What was it Gary said that was so funny? 'The girl in the Hathaway Bra.' That's me. I've lost a boob. The girl in the Hathaway Bra.*

She woke up frequently in the dark mornings at two or three and she would feel an unspecified anxiety. And she would feel, *Oh, something bad has happened.* And she would become aware of discomfort on her left side. And then she would remember, *My God, they really did it. They took off the old boob. Jesus Christ, did that really happen to me? That's really too bad. That was a really good bod I had there. It was really nice and now it isn't. Now it will never be the kind of body that anyone would go out of his way to see. In fact they'd go out of their way not to see it. Nobody is going to say, 'Boy, I can't wait to see her with her clothes off.' Never. Never. Nobody is going to say that.*

Waves of self-pity, like nausea, rolled over her. She had to fight it off. She talked to herself. *Wait a minute, you goddamned fool. What does that mean compared to the luck, the total luck, don't talk about bad luck, the total good luck, the wonderfulness of being told that you're free of cancer and you have a life ahead and you don't have to have radiology and chemotherapy and have your hair fall out. Think about that, you jerk. Concentrate on that.*

And she would fight off the self-pity and work on the feelings when they came, and they came often at two in the morning, when she felt very vulnerable. It was a solitary battle and one of the hardest kind, for it had no audience. The feelings came and she didn't know what to do with them except to fight them off. She didn't cry. She didn't wake up nights and cry, but she thought often, *why me?*

It was not always two in the morning. Sometimes during the day or early evening something would happen to dramatize her loss and she would feel, *why me?* A week after she came home she was lying on the bed watching *The Rockford Files*. She had to lie on her back to watch, for her side was still uncomfortable and her head was at an awkward angle and she sighed. David was in the room looking for a pencil and he heard her.

"Are you feeling depressed?" he said.

"Yes, I guess so. Not in the pits of depression, you know, but kind of depressed."

"I don't understand that," he said.

"I don't mean to be snotty about this," Joan said, "but it ain't your boob that was lopped off."

"Yeah, but Mom, that's just a crummy old boob. It's not your life."

And it helped. She felt the reminder and a gratitude that he was free to give it. *That's right,* she thought. *That's right, Dave. It's good that you remind me that it is just a crummy old boob.* The boys' ease with her surgery helped. When asked by their friends they spoke of their mother's mastectomy as they would have spoken of a tonsillectomy.

One afternoon Charna Levine called. A colleague at Tufts and a friend of some years, Charna called regularly to check in and see how Joan progressed.

Always Joan said bright and up-tempo things when Charna called.

"How are things?"

"Oh fine, good. I went back to work. I told my students. It was hard, but I did pretty good."

"You know," Charna said, "you must be feeling angry about this. I know you feel good as well, and you're glad it wasn't worse. But you don't want to deny the angry feelings either."

"I know."

"You have a right to those feelings, and a right to let them out."

"I don't want to dwell forever on it."

"Of course not," Charna said, "and you shouldn't. You don't want to get obsessive about all of this. But you need to let those feelings out. You shouldn't be Pollyanna Parker about it."

For Joan that was valuable. It was not that she couldn't think of such a thing. It was that she hadn't quite articulated it. And Charna having said it gave it configuration and reality. Of course she was angry. And in the days of re-entry she talked to herself almost constantly. She stayed way inside her head. She wanted not tears but anger. And she succeeded. Less and less she thought, *Oh my poor body.* More and more she thought, *I wish this did not happen, but by God it's not going to get me.*

Ace asked her one night why she was so quiet. "Are you okay," he said. "Do you feel all right?"

"Yes. I'm okay, but I have to go inside for a while," she said. "I have to keep running this experience through until somehow it becomes part of everything. You know?"

"Would it help to talk?"

"No, I don't think so. I have to do this myself."

He shrugged. She knew his feelings were hurt slightly. He was devouringly possessive and he resented anything that shut him out. But he knew that about himself and he suppressed it when he could and he knew this time she was right and he would have to stay outside, for a short while anyway.

Chapter 26 ⁓

IT TOOK perhaps two weeks for her to come to terms with the feelings of loss. *After everything is said*, she thought, *nobody really gets all that stirred up over your big problems.* She was driving now. She still moved her left arm a little carefully, but she was in control of the little Vega and the ride was pleasant. *You reach the same level of comfortable social exchange that you had before. It's not up to other people to do that for you. I have to do that. I have to act as if everything were the same. I can't wallow and revel in my sadness and my loss. It's my problem. I better get on with my life. It was given back to me, and I better use it.*

After class, on a Wednesday in mid-May, Joan went to have lunch with Marie Rawlings. It was still a women's time for her, and the friends continued to gather.

As they sipped a glass of white wine and looked at the menu, Marie said, "I really dreaded seeing you, you know."

"I can see why you might," Joan said.

"I was afraid you might not still be Joan. If you weren't Joan I wouldn't want to see you anymore. I couldn't bear it."

"But . . .?"

"But you're still Joan," Marie said.

"Yes, I am."

"And it comes across. I wondered if you'd start going with the jackets so as not to draw attention to your breasts."

Joan smiled. "I thought of that. I thought maybe people will be grossed out seeing me in a sweater or a blouse that outlines and defines the breast."

Marie shook her head.

Joan said, "That's right. That's what I decided. If people didn't like it that was their problem. If they wanted to run around saying, 'Jesus why doesn't she wear a jacket,' they would have to deal with that. I'm going to wear what I always wore. If the world wants to figure out which side is the falsie then it can go ahead."

"There's no way to tell," Marie said.

"That's right. I like the way I look when I dress like this, and Ace likes it and I am still me. I'll dress like me."

"Yes, you are," Marie said. "And it is such a relief. And if you keep it up, if you keep acting like Joan and wearing the clothes that Joan wears, and you make people see that you are still you and you have not been humbled, and you're not apologetic over what's happened to you, it will be the same."

Joan drank her wine. "It's almost the same," she said. "In some ways it's better. I feel a new power in me of what I can take. Of what I can survive."

Marie said, "Let's order." And they did.

That night in bed Joan said to Ace, "There are three things left to do."

"What are the other two?" he said.

"Getting a little randy, are we?" Joan said.

"It has now been five weeks and two days, but who counts?"

"Okay, there's that. Pretty soon, I'll be okay for that. I also have to get a prosthesis and I have to show you the incision."

"How 'bout we go to a store, make out in the fitting room, and get the whole thing done at once."

"I think we better do the incision first," she said. "You want to look?"

"Only if you want me to," he said. "I don't mind looking. I think probably we ought not to have something we don't share. But I don't want to force anything on you that will hurt."

"No, it's okay, I want you to see it. I think you should. I think we should both know what this looks like. I don't want to be worrying about it. I don't want to have to be afraid you'll catch me with my bra off."

She got up and dropped her robe from her shoulders. From the waist up she wore only a bra. She unsnapped the bra behind and removed it. The scar was a bit more puckered than he had imagined. There were still some stitches.

"What do you think?" she said.

He shrugged. "It's okay. It's not an asset but it's not gross. Dan's appendix scar looks a lot worse."

"What about the imbalance?" she said.

"It's an imbalance. You got one boob and one no-boob. But it's not gross, it's just imbalanced."

"How would you feel about it when we make love?"

"It doesn't make a lot of difference. If it's up to me I think you look better with the bra on, but it isn't very significant either way."

I think I'd rather he found me just as appealing with the bra off. But who can blame him, and it isn't much, either way. There's no way you can say, 'Isn't that attractive?' I mean one boob on and one boob off. It is what it is. It certainly isn't much of a change in our relationship, and it's hardly worth thinking about.

She slid the bra back on and put the small piece of sponge

rubber she was using, back in place. "It's better on, isn't it. Then it looks like two boobs."

"Yeah," he said. "There's no way to bullshit around that. Two boobs are better than one. But you are exactly what you have always been to me. There is no way that can change."

"I know that," she said. And she meant it. "I really believe that you want me and enjoy me physically and enjoy looking at me just as you did before. But I also believe you are absolutely the only one."

"Well, we've waltzed around that before," he said. "As long as you know about me ... 'love, let us be true to one, another ...' "

"Who said that?"

"Arnold, 'Dover Beach' ...'The sea of faith was once, too, at the full.' "

"Arghh," she said.

"You're not into verse?"

"No."

They smiled, playing their game again, feeling the expanded time they had to play such games now, for the fun of the games and not to keep an upper lip stiff. *It mattered so much,* she thought. *Slowly as I work this long thing out in my head, I am discovering how much it mattered, the knowledge that he wouldn't change, that he would love me and want me and enjoy me just as he did before, and that for him I am exactly what I always was. I will be grateful for that till I die.*

"Perhaps," he said, "you might enjoy it if I were to recite the starting lineup of the nineteen forty-six Brooklyn Dodgers, including all eight guys that they tried at third base that year."

"Perhaps you would just as soon forget forever about sexual activity," she said.

It sustained me more, I think, than I knew. That and the

knowledge that the boys would be the same. That sustains beyond all else, to the ones that mean the most, I am still me.

"Okay, never mind about the Brooklyn Dodgers. What's next, the screw or the prosthesis?"

"Ugh," she said. "I hate that word."

"Which? Screw or prosthesis?"

"Prosthesis."

"Whew."

"I think of trusses and artificial limbs, and cumbersome contraptions done in black leather."

"Ah, now you're talking my language," he said.

"Not that kind of contraption, weirdo."

"Oh."

"But anyway, to answer your question. The prosthesis is next. I saw an ad in the *Globe* today. For Jodi bras."

"Yeah, I did too. I went over and checked it out. You just walk in. No appointment. They have someone who helps you get fitted."

"You went and asked about it?"

"Yeah. I asked some saleslady who looked very concerned that the Jodi bra lady wasn't there. So I said, 'That's okay, I don't need her now anyway. It's not for me, it's for my wife.' " He began to giggle. "She looked at me quite strangely and went away quickly."

"I bet they love you in stores," she said, her face bright with laughter. "Anyway, I'm going over tomorrow and get one."

"Want me to come?"

"No. Jude will go with me. I'm not completely comfortable with you seeing the incision again. And someone has to go in the fitting room and they might not let you in."

"There would have to be a fair number of salesladies to keep me out."

"Anyway, I'm completely comfortable with Jude. She's seen the incision and all. I won't be embarrassed with her. So tomorrow she and I will go."

"Do they make them in black lace with cat faces over the nipples?" he said.

"Animal."

Chapter 27 ⟿

THURSDAY MORNING after the kids were off to school Joan said to Judy Marsh, "You gotta come with me. I gotta get this over with. If you come with me it will be funny. If I go by myself I may cry a lot."

Judy said, "Let's go now so we can be there when the store opens and we won't have a bunch of people standing around listening when we are asking at the bra counter."

Judy drove. In the car they discussed phrasing.

"Just say, 'I'd like to see a Jodi bra, please,'" Judy said.

"And what if she says, 'What's a Jodi bra?'" Joan said.

"Then you say, 'I've had a mastectomy.'"

"And what if she says, 'What's a mastectomy?'" Joan said.

"Then you call her an asshole," Judy said.

"I guess we'll play it by ear," Joan said.

At the bra counter Joan said to the saleswoman, "Excuse me, I understand you sell Jodi bras."

"Yes, we do."

"I'd like to look at some Jodi bras specifically for the left side."

Beside her Jude murmured, "Nice phrasing."

"Shut up, Jude, it's the best I can think of."

The saleswoman said, "I couldn't possibly help you with a Jodi bra, but our surgical fitter will."

Joan looked at Judy. Judy formed the words "surgical fitter" silently and raised her eyebrows. The saleslady went to get the surgical fitter.

"What the hell," Joan said, "is a surgical fitter? Is she going to operate?"

Judy said, "I bet it gets worse."

The surgical fitter was a small fat lady with her hair dyed black and a strong Bronx accent. She appeared to be about fifty-five. She wore a lot of jewelry, and the smell of her perfume was strong and inexpensive.

"Darling," she said with a big smile, "I am here to help you."

"Listen," Joan said, "what I need is a little something to shove in the left side to even things off."

"Come right along with me, dear," the surgical fitter said. "We'll go in the fitting room, and you can take off your blouse and bra and I'll surgically fit you."

Judy made a small noise next to Joan. The surgical fitter looked slightly annoyed.

"Right away, we've got a problem," Joan said. "I don't want to go in the fitting room and take off my blouse and bra. I feel a little silly about it, but I am just not ready to bare the bod to anyone but my friend," Joan pointed to Judy. The surgical fitter did not look at Judy.

"But, honey," the surgical fitter said, "think of me as your doctor." *I am inclined to think of my doctor as my doctor,* Joan thought, *and I tend to think of this person as someone who's going to sell me a falsie. Still, she does this for a living and I don't want to dump on her.* "I appreciate that you're trying to help me," Joan said, "but the best way for you to do that is to recognize that I'm a little, uh, eccentric. So you just show me a Jodi bra or two and Jude and I will try them out."

The surgical fitter went somewhat glumly to get a Jodi bra. Several old ladies had gathered at the bra counter to buy a Bali bra and stopped to watch. The surgical fitter returned with an apparatus that looked like a suspension bridge. "Jesus Christ," Joan said. Jude was contorted with suppressed laughter. "Joan," she murmured, "I'm going to wet my pants."

The bra had side panels nearly five inches across with thick heavy straps. "Ma'am," Joan said to the surgical fitter, "that bra is obviously meant to contain undulating, pendulous breasts." Joan pointed to her chest. "Could you look at my terrific chest and my magnificent bod and see that I don't have a lot of equipment there? I mean I never wore a bra like that in my life. I will not start wearing one now."

"Honey, it is meant to hold the Jodi form," the surgical fitter said.

"You mean Jodi only makes forms for huge-breasted women?"

"Oh no, we make them all sizes."

"Well, see if you can find one that would be maybe an A cup size or A form or whatever you call it."

"Certainly. I'll just take a look in the back."

She left. The other ladies completed their transactions for normal bras, but two of them lingered, looking at stockings, waiting to see how things worked out.

Joan said to Judy, "Isn't this thrilling?"

"This woman may be the biggest asshole in the western world," Judy said.

"I wouldn't limit her that way," Joan said.

The surgical fitter returned with a lump of siliconish-looking material shaped somewhat like a breast. She put it on the counter and they all stared at it. It looked like a large translucent grapefruit. In bra terms it was at least an E cup. The surgical fitter said, "There."

Jude's voice was shaking. "Joan . . ." she said.

Joan said, "I don't mean to be rude, but look at me. Don't you think if I were to shove that great rubbery thing inside my bra it would overpower the other side. I mean that's very large, and I'm not very large."

The surgical fitter was disappointed. She said, "Well, sweetheart, if you would just step into the fitting room I could fit you properly."

"Why can't we compromise," Joan said. "Judy and I will go into the fitting room and you can hand things into the fitting room and we'll do it that way."

The surgical fitter reluctantly agreed to that. This was not the way she'd been trained. She picked up the great rubber grapefruit and the great huge bra, and led Joan and Judy to the fitting room. Joan and Judy went in. Joan took off her blouse. "Now," she said through the curtain, "you just hand me that grapefruity thing."

Joan took out the old foam falsie she had been wearing, and the gauze padding and shoved the grapefruit inside her bra. Judy's eyes filled with tears and she leaned helplessly against the wall of the fitting room. "Joan," she said, gasping for breath, "I'm going to be hysterical."

The left side of her chest stuck out aggressively, twice the size of her real breast. She opened the curtain, her bra in place and said to the surgical fitter. "What do you think?"

"It's a little big," the surgical fitter said.

"Yes," Joan said, "let's try a smaller size. The surgical fitter brought a D. It was too big. She brought a C, it was too big. She brought a B. It was too big. "She's not a quitter, is she," Judy said.

What seemed to Joan maybe an A½ size was about right.

"Now," said the surgical fitter, "you'll need a new bra." She looked very scornfully at Joan's old bra. She had been wearing it every day because it was comfortable, taking it off at night to run it through the washer and dryer. The bra looked tired and gray. "I'm here only to help you, honey. I've helped a lot of women. I've fitted a lot of women and they come back and tell me that they went out into the store to show Hubby, and Hubby says to them, 'Sweetheart, you've never looked so even.'"

Jesus Christ, if that's my goal in life, Joan thought, *I am in severe trouble.*

Judy said, "I think she'd be better off with a regular bra. You know, a Playtex, or a Rogers Formfit, or whatever."

Wearily the surgical fitter went back out of the fitting room and wearily she returned with a Rogers Formfit. "Ah," Joan said, "now we're talking about the kind of bra I wear." The surgical fitter stepped out of the fitting room and Joan took off her bra and slipped into the new one.

"Look at that," Judy said, "a regular, ordinary bra, like the ladies wear in the dressing room at Loehmann's."

Joan shoved the form into the left cup and adjusted the bra. "There I am," she said.

Judy said, "That looks terrific."

And it did. With the bra on Joan looked perfectly normal. Perhaps a quarter of an inch of scar showed at the V of the bra, but otherwise there was no sign that she was not as she had been. The prosthesis moved with her; she felt it and it felt like her. She could be bumped, hugged, poked at, and no one would know the difference.

The surgical fitter was pleased. "It's puncture-proof, darling." *Puncture-proof,* Joan thought, *I wonder what she thinks my sex life is like.* "And guaranteed five years. There's no worry about this for five years, darling." Joan felt a flash of indulgent humor. *Five years,* she thought, *well, Christ, in five years this thing will grow back.* That was followed by a brief stab of depression. *No, it won't. It's gone forever. If this thing does last in its puncture-proof purity for five years I'll have to come back and go through this again.* There was always that part of her which perceived the operation as temporary, which rejected forever.

Joan paid, and she and Judy went out of the store. "Joan," Judy said. "I don't think I can go through this every five years."

"There's got to be a better way," Joan said.

"I'll find out some places that do this sort of thing, at the hospital," Jude said. "I know there are easier ways. Longwood Pharmacy in Boston, I think. They make a pocket in your bra and everything."

"Do you think they employ a surgical fitter?" Joan said.

"Oh God, I hope not," Jude said.

Epilogue ~⌒

A FRIDAY NIGHT, six weeks to the day since she discovered the first hint of breast cancer, Joan said to Ace, "Don't think this is going to be fun, because it isn't. But it's time to resume sexual activity."

"You sensuous bitch," he said.

"I mean it. Don't think of this as a fun time. Think of this as a sort of experiment. We very carefully try it out and see if it's okay yet. It's not going to be a big treat."

"It's probably won't be much worse than the cold showers I've been taking."

"Okay. Here's what we'll do. We'll pretend we're very old people and we'll do the whole thing very gingerly. Very carefully."

"Tough, but oh so gentle," Ace said.

"Maybe," Joan said. "But the weight. The two hundred twenty pounds tends to worry me."

"I can take most of it on my arms," Ace said. "Like doing a push-up. . . . Or a push-in, as the case may be."

"Cute," Joan said. "That's very cute, Bob. You keep being cute while I go and suit up as we say."

Joan went into the bathroom. "Suit up?" Ace said after her.

I'll have to wear my bra, she thought. *What else? Anything? How much of the bod do I show? How about my robe? To be naked with just a bra seems somehow too naked or too seductive, when I am in fact unseductive. Or maybe I am unseductive because I have but one boob. A naked woman in a bra tends to emphasize the bra. That's why all those bra ads are like that. I don't want that. I'll go with the robe.* She emerged from the bathroom, wearing her green terry-cloth robe with the vertical rainbow stripes.

"Terry cloth is nice," Ace said, "but actually I'm more into leather, and maybe some silver chains."

"Shut up," she said. "I've given this a lot of thought. This is it."

"Well, it's better than on our wedding night when you wore the goddamned hairnet."

"If you'll recall," she said, "it was called a ravishing hairnet and it had little rosebuds on it."

"Yeah."

"First thing we do," she said, "is, we practice."

"Oh hell, Joan, I'm not that rusty."

"Never mind, we practice. I am very protective of my left side and you are very big and active."

"Remember the time just before we got married when you'd been fitted for a diaphragm and you were afraid that you wouldn't be able to put it in right, so you wanted to practice?"

"Um-hm."

"And you put it in on the floor in your mother's living room and I had to wait in the den in case it got stuck and you couldn't get it out?"

"Well, for crissake. The time I tried it in the doctor's office it slipped out of my hand and flew up in the air and hit the ceiling."

"Yeah, I guess you needed the practice. How's this?" He supported his weight on his arms.

"That's okay," she said, "that's good. But what about you? Is that comfortable?"

"Oh, don't worry about me."

"No, is it?"

"Yeah, that's fine. You know how powerful I am. I could stay like this thirty or forty seconds with no problem."

"Ace!"

"It's fine. It really is."

"Good. Now, no touching the chest."

"Okay by me. I tend to forget which side is which and I'd feel like a real jerk getting off on a falsie."

"Getting off on a falsie? That's what I like about you, Bob, you're so sensitive."

He kissed her.

"How do you think it's going so far?" he said.

"That wasn't too bad," she said.

Carefully, gently, thoughtfully, they made love. Part of Joan analyzed and recorded. *That's okay. That doesn't hurt. This is all right. By Christ, we're doing okay . . . I wonder if he minds. I wonder if he can tell that one boob is a falsie? Does he feel the difference? Is he fantasizing some zoftig two-boobed lovely? A complete woman? I hope not. I don't blame him but I hope he isn't.*

"You okay?" he said.

"Yes," she said.

He's concentrating on what's left. She thought. *Not what's gone.*

Afterward they were quiet in the dark, lying side by side on their backs, holding hands. Upstairs the boys were asleep. From his place under the drape the dog made his sleeping sounds.

They were home. They were in the good place. And they would be there tomorrow.

"What do you think?" she said. "What do you think about the one boob?"

He raised one eyebrow in the dark and sucked his cheeks in and said, "Frankly, my dear, I don't give a damn."